THE BOOK ON BIOFEEDBACK
HOW TO REACH
HEALTH & WELLNESS IN ONE MINUTE!

DR. THÉRÈSE MICHEL-MANSOUR (PH.D.)

RAYMOND AARON, NEW YORK TIMES
BEST-SELLING AUTHOR

ISBN: 978-1-77277-031-5

PUBLISHED BY:
10-10-10 PUBLISHING
MARKHAM, ON
CANADA

Disclaimer

The information in this book does not constitute medical advice. Readers are advised to seek professional medical assistance in the event that they are suffering from any medical problem.

Dedication

I dedicate this book to my late sister Nadine (Michel) Sharawy and to the "new generation" of loving, spirited and accomplished family members including: Ashlin, Caitlin, Christiane, Danielle, Evelyn, Justin, Mark, Mathew and Natalie.

Acknowledgements

My absolute and most tender thanks go to my husband, Kamal Mansour. His love and support throughout our marriage is an essential cornerstone of my recovery. He is an essential part of this book and any other endeavours I have undertaken. I wish to articulate my warmest gratitude to my son, Mark James, whose wisdom, integrity, impeccable work ethics and intellectual savvy are matched only by his humility and his patience. To Christiane Marie, my sweet daughter, I can truly say she nurtures and inspires me daily to fight back!

My journey towards wellness has lasted for years and yet I feel it has just begun. Throughout it all, my family, constitutes my undying supporters. I wish to dedicate this book to the memory and lasting legacy of my late sister, Nadine. An immensely accomplished, gifted and loving person. She remains an inspiration of dignity to our family. My deepest admiration and love go to my younger sister Sherine. She has *always* provided me with unwavering strength and unconditional love. To her I owe immeasurable gratitude. To Hani Michel, my brother who always "teased me" but never failed me in his love or sweet predisposition, I remain forever grateful. To my whole family, especially my nieces and nephews, and their significant others, I wish to express my fondest gratitude for their "warmth" and "spirited ways" that cheered me on! Thank you.

This book would not be possible without the significant contribution of several academic and medical professionals I have come to respect and admire throughout my career. To the late Dr. Frederick Ivor Case (Professor, University of Toronto),

I offer my deepest and most sincere thanks for mentoring me and believing in me throughout: "grand merci, mon cher ami!" To Professor Janet Paterson (University of Toronto), I present my warmest regards and gratitude for her solid support and friendship during my academic career.

A few very special medical professionals I have encountered on my path to wellness have greatly inspired me and, by extension, the writing of this book. I wish to express my gratitude to each and every one of them. I shall do so in the chronological order of their intervention in my recovery.

I wish to express my deepest thanks to Dr. Walter Himmel (Canada) for his passion for investigative, "avant-garde" research on "Fatigue" back in 2004. In my view, his ethics for research, merely out of interest, combined with his patient care, define him as an outstanding practitioner.

I wish to convey my utmost regard and respect to Dr. Jacob Teitelbaum, (United States), for his pioneering and ground-breaking research on Chronic Fatigue Syndrome which, even today, continues to inspire practitioners and patients alike.

My utmost admiration and gratitude go to Dr. Marvin Sponaugle (United-States). His inspirational wisdom and expertise regarding the new age real threat of "Toxicity" is, for me, matched only by his holistic, cutting edge healing protocol. Indeed, this book is a testament to the efficacy of his protocol and intervention in my case. I am deeply grateful to him!

Last but not least, I wish to express my sincere gratitude to Dr. George Grant (Canada). He ushered me into a new chapter in my endeavour, the Biofeedback Technology, which informs considerably this book. His multi-dimensional expertise in the medical field coupled with his passion for "teaching" are a testament to his practice and prolific publications. I thank him for sharing generously with me his personal and professional experience.

To my co-author, Mr. Raymond Aaron (Canada), I express my deepest admiration for his astonishing publishing success and brilliant mind. I am very fortunate to have the rare chance to co-author this book with him! I look forward to its launch!

In closing, I extend my kindest regards to the whole 10-10-10 Publishing team for their professional support.

Foreword

Much of Western Allopathic methods of diagnosis depends on invasive procedures involving radiation, expense and potential side effects.

In this book, Dr. Thérèse Michel-Mansour introduces the reader to the Biofeedback scan, an accurate medical device, non-invasive, safe health and wellness total body assessment. In less than 2 minutes, the scan's 35 organs and systems panels reveal the health status of every organ. It is possible for any person to optimize their health through lifestyle changes and natural supplements.

Dr. Thérèse joined our team at www.academyofwellness.com and has contributed immensely in the assessment of clients, corporations and non-profit organizations using Quantum Biofeedback.

Dr. Thérèse is a life-long learner with a passion to help her clients improve their lifestyle habits, recommending health awareness and natural supplements to help them live healthy to 101+.

Prevention over intervention is a principle that can be applied to anyone of any background. *The Book on Biofeedback* will help you to understand and incorporate the use of this non-invasive and accurate device to thrive to 101+ years of age with vibrant health.

Dr. George Grant, Ph.D., IMD, M.Sc. "The Caring Doctor"
Best selling Author of 10 books. Former Consultant for Health Canada, FDA & CDC.

www.academyofwellness.com ; www.your101ways.com

About the Author

Dr. Thérèse Michel-Mansour was awarded "Best Thesis of the Year Award" in 1992, by the Department of French Studies, University of Toronto.

Her book entitled *La portée esthétique du signe dans le texte maghrébin* (Paris: Publisud, 1994), is considered a cornerstone of the "Principles of Aesthetics" of the Maghreb Novel and is sold worldwide. She published in *The Encyclopedia of the Novel* (1998) and is the author of thirteen refereed papers published in academic works and reviews.

Former Assistant Professor at the University of Toronto, Université de Montréal and Professor at Seneca College, Dr. Michel-Mansour remains an active member of "Conseil International d'Études Francophones". She presents her research in universities around the world including Canada, the United States, Europe, North Africa, South America and the Mauritius.

She is a public speaker, multilingual, passionate and creative person whose message is: "Wellness is Bio Awareness"!

Dr. Michel-Mansour is a Biofeedback Therapist and practises in the Toronto Area.

About the Book

This book is based on the author's personal journey to health and wellness, coupled with her professional training and experience.

Her recommendations are inspired by her discovery of alternative medical healing protocols, one of which is the **Biofeedback Quantum Resonance Analyzer** medical device.

The author's conviction is that "Awareness" of one's body (bio) state, followed by "Action" pursuant to the discovery of that state, ultimately lead to an "Awesome" optimization of one's health. The examples used by the author demonstrate how *pre-emption* through early detection of body toxicity level, of nutrient deficiency and/or predisposition to common illnesses, is key to wellness enhancement.

Given the accuracy, sensitivity and the non-invasive nature of the bio-scan, the author maintains most health issues are reversible through the use of highly absorbable natural supplements (95% absorption rate) and the reduction of toxic exposure.

Dr. Michel-Mansour guides you throughout your journey back to optimal health.

Preamble

This book is divided into two parts.

Part I includes Chapters 1-7. They primarily introduce the Quantum Resonance Magnetic Analyzer as a medical device. The chapters demonstrate its application in order to enhance existing health issues and / or pre-empt their onset using physiological markers.

Part II includes Chapters 8-10. This part seeks to complete the bio-awareness focus by integrating the psychological and spiritual dimensions of a healthy existence. Balancing stress with self-healing and self-actualization elevates our existence to a higher sphere, that of the spiritual.

Table of Contents

Introduction

What determines your health state and longevity is the degree to which you minimize your level of toxicity. As you grow older two things happen: your body has been exposed to free radicals longer and your environment becomes progressively more toxic. Free radicals are everywhere: food, water, air, pesticides, contaminants, GMOs even UV rays.

The first step is to acknowledge that, every day you survive, you increase your exposure to toxicity. Realizing that asthma, skin conditions, insomnia, hair loss, memory loss, arthritis...etc. are not "normal aging" symptoms, but are symptoms of the increasing inflammation in your body due to free radical activity, is the initial phase on the road to recovery.

The second step is to identify your symptoms' root cause through your bio-scan and to respond to the root cause with nutritional health. The Biofeedback Scan is a non-invasive, highly accurate quantum-medicine device which takes 60 seconds to let "your body speak to you". It measures the health of your circulatory, cardiovascular, endocrine, digestive and intestinal systems amongst others.

The third step is to act upon the information provided to you by the bio-scan. You owe it to yourself to lead the way to "Health and Wellness" with your bio-scan, where Wellness is Bio Awareness!!

PART ONE

CHAPTER 1
HOW BIOFEEDBACK SCAN CAN
IMPROVE YOUR HEALTH

"Biofeedback" is defined as the process or mechanism through which the body (bio) reveals information about itself (feedback). The Biofeedback Scan is a device that allows your body to "speak back to you". The Quantum Resonance Magnetic Analyzer is a hi-tech innovation device, which is related to medical bioinformatics engineering. It is based on quantum (infinite) medicine. It scientifically analyzes the human cells' magnetic field activity which is then processed by the device and presented in panels referring to various body functions and systems (see the Bio-Scan Charts video at www.biofeedbackbook.com). By holding the sensor of the analyzer in the palm of your hand for *one minute*, the sensor detects, through your palm, the cells' activity (watch One Minute Bio-Scan on www.biofeedbackbook.com).

The cells in your body are continually growing, developing, differentiating, regenerating and dying. There are about twenty-five million cells in your body dividing and multiplying per second. During this process, which is detected during the one minute scan, electromagnetic waves are radiating outward constantly and are captured by the sensor and transmitted to the scanner. The energy and speed of the electrons' electromagnetic waves variation are detected by the sensor and reflect the specific states of the human body as healthy, sub-healthy or diseased state.

The biofeedback scan is a comprehensive, individualized health consulting medical device. It is non-invasive, simple, quick, economical and, most importantly, it is accurate. It is comprised of thirty-five panels offering a considerable range of body functions. It includes the cardiovascular and cerebrovascular functions, the endocrine, immune, circulatory, respiratory, gastrointestinal systems as well as the nutritional levels of vitamins, minerals, amino acids, human toxins, and allergens…etc.

A glimpse at the chart entitled *Cardiovascular and Cerebrovascular Data Analysis* provided in Table 1[1] provides an illustrative example. For a more comprehensive look at the thirty five panels of the scan, please visit "Panel Video" on www.biofeedbackbook.com. Thirty five panels constitute a comprehensive array of vital information, in real time, about your body's performance and needs, all literally at your fingertips! Each panel is color-coded and includes various entries. Each entry provides the Normal Range to which you compare your Actual Measurement Value given (refer to Table 1). An entry in any given panel will guide you in "reading" your body's information. By simply comparing your "Actual" value to the "Normal Range" you will see how your body is performing (watch Read Your Measurement at www.biofeedbackbook.com).

So why use the bio-scan? The scan has multiple advantages. One of the most valued advantages is that it is sensitive and precise enough to detect early onset of disease, allowing you to

---

[1] Please refer to the end of Chapter 7 for Table 1. From this point forward in the text, D.A. refers to "Data Analysis". Reference to video titles throughout the chapters refer to videos number 1-8 on www.biofeedbackbook.com.

pre-empt further deterioration of your health and/or to intervene in order to reverse and correct most health issues. For example, if you are unaware that you have "insulin resistance" (when cells do not respond to insulin prompting to allow glucose to be absorbed by them), a condition considered a precursor to diabetes, or that your "bone mineral density" levels are inching towards osteoporosis, that information, revealed through the scan, will alert and empower you to reverse these tendencies.

Another real and effective advantage is that, once you are scanned, you will receive a compositive scan (or summary) of your scan results via email the same day. Your Actual Measurement Value compared to the Normal Range value is given in a three decimal point figure for each entry (see the video entitled Values on www.biofeedbackbook.com). Your follow-up scan three months later will surprise you as it is readily comparable, entry for entry, with your first scan.

As for accuracy, the bio scan is highly accurate and comparable to other more invasive and time-consuming methods of testing. Most valuable, however, is the *comprehensive component* of the whole body performance measured by the bio-scan (visit www.biofeedbackbook.com/ Comprehensive Body Scan).

So how can the comprehensive component of your bio-scan improve your health? Since all systems in the body are interconnected and are interdependent, revealing their connections, or identifying their ripple effect, is a vital advantage. For example, consider, very briefly, the Ancient Egyptian medical model. The highest priest, trained in the sciences of human anatomy and in the spiritual realms, was the medical advisor. His first task consisted of overseeing specialists under him. He was responsible for synthesizing all their findings about the patient's condition. He disposed of all available findings and made "connections", "links" between their findings; then, and only then, was he able to provide the best advice to the patient.

In a similar way the bio-scan dispenses information concerning your whole body. With the guidance of the therapist you are enabled to understand your body from "inside out" as a "whole", dynamic, not static, unit. Every function and every measurement is interdependent or co-dependent upon a series of other functions or measurements, and their connection helps you identify the "root" cause of your health concern. In turn, this means that you can address your condition and not the symptom!

For example, you might have a high level of Blood Viscosity indicated in the *Cardiovascular and Cerebrovascular D.A.* You may assume that this blood "thickness" can be addressed with a blood thinner. This is probably a reductive (simple but non-productive) solution. However, should you discover simultaneously, during your scan consultation, that the viscosity is related to a high Blood Fat, or cholesterol level, measured in the same panel, your approach to the solution may be, then, very different.

Further, other panels will confirm or refute the blood fat / blood viscosity hypothesis. One such panel is the *Blood Lipids D.A.* which measures your total cholesterol and breaks it down into the High Density Lipoprotein (HDL-C) and the Low Density Lipoprotein (LDL). Each measurement reflects your blood fat cholesterol components into the "good" and the "bad" cholesterol. When you compare these numbers to the "Normal Range" indicated, you will be able to either confirm or refute the cholesterol issue, as it relates to your blood viscosity (watch the video on The Blood Viscosity Mystery on www.biofeedbackbook.com).

Also, quite possibly, there is no cholesterol issue behind the "blood viscosity". Another root cause is also measured during the scan. It is your level of toxicity measured through your response to toxin exposure to various toxic agents. The link between blood thickness and toxins is simple. Toxins that we inhale, ingest or come in physical contact with through our skin cause our body to react to them. The body does so by releasing high levels of histamine in our blood. High histamine level leads to blood thickening or viscosity.

There are four panels in the scan compositive that address your toxicity and your allergic reaction to some of the most common toxins in the environment. By examining your results you can very possibly identify the root cause of your blood viscosity. The *Human Toxin D.A.* measures your body's reaction to separate categories of toxins such as Electromagnetic Radiation, Tobacco/Nicotine, and Toxic Pesticide Residue. *The Heavy Metal D.A.* specifically tests your levels of the heavy metals you are reacting to including: Lead, Cadmium, Arsenic, Chrome and Mercury.

Equally revealing are two more panels the *Skin D.A.* and the *Allergen D.A.* which determine the specific products and materials to which you are reacting (see video on Toxicity Panels). If you become aware of the link between your allergic response to specific toxins and your blood viscosity, it is possible that your approach to treatment may be considerably different. Now that you are informed about the root cause of the symptom, you may choose to address the former not the latter. The bio-scan highlights the link between symptoms and condition, enabling you to discern the root cause.

Another example is that of cholesterol which, according to statistics, is no longer a middle-age condition but is seen more so in younger adults. The link between elevated cholesterol level, measured under *Blood Lipids D.A.*, insulin level in *Pancreatic Function D.A.*, and vascular resistance measured in *Cardiovascular D.A.*, has been medically proven. The body's insulin secretion controls the fat, glucose and protein metabolism which, if not metabolised, may in turn cause hardening of the arteries. Ultimately arteriosclerosis leads to vascular resistance, a form of blood pressure, be it mild or severe.

Nevertheless, should you discover early on that you have "insulin resistance", you may intervene before any of the above takes place. For example, the bio-scan measures your insulin resistance in more than one way. How? We know that insulin secretion by the pancreas rises after eating carbohydrates, rich foods, sweets or fruits. The insulin prompts the cells to allow glucose in, to be absorbed and converted into energy. Should that signal fail, for some reason, the glucose is stored in the body. Insulin resistance occurs when the cells resist the insulin's orders as the pancreas keeps on secreting more insulin. However, once the pancreas can no longer keep up with the requirement for more insulin, blood glucose levels rise. This is a common cause of type 2 diabetes. How can the bio-scan detect this predisposition earlier? The *Blood Sugar D.A.* and the *Liver Function D.A.* are instrumental in identifying the "resistance" and in guiding you.

The *Blood Sugar D.A.* measures your Coefficient of Insulin Secretion in the blood, the Blood Sugar Coefficient and the Urine Sugar Coefficient. All three readings determine whether you have insulin imbalance (the insulin secretion is too high or too low) and whether that imbalance is significant enough to cause deposit of sugar in blood or urine. The second panel *Liver*

Function D.A. tests your Protein Metabolism and your Liver Fat Content which would corroborate the first finding of insulin imbalance.

Similarly, should you be taking statins medication to lower your cholesterol, you should monitor your Coenzyme Q10 as statins lower that vital coenzyme. Even more revealing to you is perhaps the discovery that, even though you have been supplementing with Coenzyme Q10, your level, according to your measurement, is below the normal range according to the *Coenzyme D.A.* This finding would point to a poor *absorption* of your Coenzyme Q10 supplement. Nutrients absorption and digestion, which involve the gastrointestinal tract, are necessary processes to convert food and nutrients into energy and release wastes (refer to Chapter 5). How various nutrients are digested and how the breakdown of products traverse (cross) the cells lining, the small intestine to reach the blood stream and to be used by the other cells of the body, is a very complex process. The *Freiburg Study* commissioned in Germany in 2014, demonstrates, in clinical tests, how *absorption* impacts the end result of nutrients tested (visit www.freiburgstudy.com). However, ensuring your levels are optimized is difficult without specific measurements offered by the bio-scan.

How else can a scan help you reach and maintain optimum health? Oxygenation of every cell in your body is a must. Scientists proved that a diseased cell lacks proper oxygen absorption. This coefficient is measured in the *Lung Function D.A.* As well, you might be surprised to learn that shallow breathing (i.e. breathing from the chest) is the precursor to lower oxygenation of the whole body, specifically of your brain cells tissue. Belly breathing, that is drawing your breath from deep within the belly, allows air to travel all the way to your brain cells, the highest point in the body and therefore the furthest to reach. It takes practise to belly-breathe but it is worth the effort.

Practise 10 breaths every hour, thereby training your brain to do so more automatically on regular basis.

In the next few chapters you shall be able to appreciate the many beneficial facets of a one minute bio-scan that can make a considerable difference in your approach to optimizing your state of health and wellness.

CHAPTER 2
TOXICITY A SERIOUS THREAT TO YOU

When you know you are not "feeling great" but there is no medical evidence to support your claim, chances are your body is too toxic. You can rely on the bio-scan to allow you to account for your present state of health.

Since our body produces its own load of toxins and free radicals (refer to Chapter 3), it is essential to reduce outside factors which increase our toxic load. Information and intervention then become key to reducing your toxin exposure. As the body uses nutrients for energy to detoxify itself, it is necessary to combine proper nutrients with strategies to damage control toxins' effect.

So what are human toxins? A toxin is a poisonous substance produced within the living cells or organisms in the human body. Also, toxins are part and parcel of our daily environment. They are capable of causing disease on contact with or by absorption by the body tissues. They also interact with biological macromolecules such as enzymes or cellular receptors.

Where are toxins? They are everywhere. There are two broad categories of toxins. Synthetic toxicants are created by artificial processes. For instance, arsenic is used to strengthen alloys of copper, lead in car batteries and electronic devices, as well, as in pesticides, herbicides and insecticides. The second category includes environmental toxins: plastics, food and water supply contaminants. Industrial smokestacks are the main culprits. They disseminate dioxins (from plastics, pesticides and other chemicals) and PCB's in the air, rain, soil, food, water, plants, animals and humans. Plastics and their outgas, for example, leak into all our food and drink supply.

How do toxins harm you? Since scientists and researchers confirmed that humans cannot metabolize nor eliminate toxins, toxins have a cumulative effect on your body. Consider, for example, what you may be inhaling day and night in your home or office: formaldehyde in insulation material, carpet out-gases (containing over 200 chemicals) and house cleaning agents... etc. Once in the body they damage hormone receptors, which leads to loss of energy and sex drive. They damage our brain chemistry leading to disability and hyperactivity. They accumulate in organs and trigger cancer of the prostate, lungs, thyroids and auto-immune diseases.

The longer you live the more elevated is your toxic level. A high toxic level or, *oxidative stress* is related to the inflammation caused by free radical activity (see Chapter 3) and their damage to your cells. Oxidative stress depends on two factors. The first is your body's ability to detoxify using the liver, the lymph nodes, the kidney etc. This is a major factor, since no two individuals detoxify their body in exactly the same way nor to the same degree. The second is your ability to reduce your exposure and or consumption of toxic products thereby reducing your toxic load.

How can your bio-scan help you with your toxins load? The bio-scan has six toxin-specific panels divided into two groups. The first group, determines your body's toxicity level with respect to major toxins. The second group measures your body's coping abilities with respect to these toxins.

The first group of panels consists of the *Human Toxin D.A.*, *Heavy Metals D.A.* and *Allergen D.A.* They depict the specific toxin group and its toxic level in your body (see video on Toxicity Panels in www.biofeedbackbook.com). The second group consists of three panels: *Liver Function D.A*, *Basic Physical Quality D.A.* and *Skin D.A.* They measure your body's coping level by pointing to its strengths or weaknesses.

The *Human Toxin D.A.* panel categorizes and measures your own body toxins load under the following criteria: Heavy Metals, Stimulating Beverage, Electromagnetic Radiation, Nicotine and Toxic Pesticide Residue. While it would be near impossible to test for the over one thousand toxins in our environment, the above categories do give a reasonable indication of your toxic load. The first sub category Heavy Metals group will be further subdivided into five specific heavy metals, particularly the ones most common in concentration in our environment: Lead, Cadmium, Arsenic, Chrome and Mercury. We shall return to this sub group shortly in this chapter.

It is worthwhile to briefly comment on the *Human Toxin D.A.* categories. The entry Stimulating Beverage can be misleading at first as people generally associate stimulating drinks with coffee or tea. However, this category refers equally to forms of sugars as stimulants (fructose, glucose, sucrose etc.), to certain color pigment, carbonated water and carbon dioxide, all of which have no nutritional benefit, but are mild toxicants. Electromagnetic Radiation is recognized today as the number one major pollutant in the world, being ranked before sewage, waste and noise pollutants. While the health hazard of nicotine measured in the Tobacco/ Nicotine panel is well known, the information is not always a deterrent since nicotine is addictive. Fortunately, second hand smoke is included in this category and can thankfully alert non-smokers to their exposure risk. Toxic Pesticide Residue (elaborated further in Chapters 3 & 4) can alter our hormone secretion and is impossible to eliminate from the body. Each of these sub-categories is measured by the bio-scan and your toxic level for each is measured precisely. Awareness of their existence and their load in your body can allow you to address them specifically.

Take a moment now to consider the threat to your health, due to exposure to the heavy metals above. Identification and proper response are key. Toxins largely destroy the myelin sheath (a protective nerve cover) which makes up 80% of the brain mass. They are released in the blood stream and increase the histamine production in the body, an inflammation marker, which can thicken the blood as discussed in Chapter 1. Demyelation of the brain cells can affect the four-second memory which builds our data memory bank. They also tax the liver which, in turn, becomes less effective in detoxifying your body.

In the *Heavy Metals D.A.*, the bio-scan tests for five major heavy metals. Lead, for example, is considered a metabolic poison, which means that it inhibits some basic enzyme functions (Chapters 3 & 5). Lead reacts with selenium and sulfur diminishing their ability to protect against free radical damage. When lead is present in the body, it can damage the heart, kidneys, liver and nervous system. Sources of lead exposure include lead-based paints, ceramic glazes, lead crystal dishes, glass ware, leaded gasoline…etc. Water supplied through lead piping is another significant source.

Cadmium is naturally present in the environment. It replaces the body's stores of the essential mineral zinc in the liver and kidneys. Its toxicity threatens the health of your body by weakening your immune system. It causes decreased production of T-lymphocytes (T cells), the key white blood cells that protect your body by destroying foreign invaders and cancer cells. Because it is mostly stored in the kidneys and liver, excessive exposure to cadmium can lead to kidney disease and serious liver damage.

Arsenic is a highly poisonous metallic element found in a wide variety of sources including pesticides, laundry aids, smog, tobacco, smoke, kelp, table salt, beer, seafood and even drinking water. It primarily affects the lungs, skin, kidney and liver.

Chrome exposure is mostly inhaled and can lead to respiratory cancer. Metal furnishing, leather tanning and dye products are mostly responsible. But chromium is also present in our water supply. It accumulates mainly in the liver, kidney and endocrine glands.

Mercury is one of the most toxic metals even more so than lead. This poison is found in our soil, water, food supply, fungicides and pesticides. It is also widely used in cosmetics, dental fillings, fabric softeners, batteries, industrial instruments, inks (used by painters and tattooists), in some medications, some paints, polishes, plastics, solvents and wood preservatives. According to the World Health Organization the most significant source of mercury exposure comes from amalgam dental fillings. They are a prime source of exposure. Mercury reaches brain cells and the central nervous system. Its impact on our body has been heavily documented. Suffice it to say that it can cause anyone to lose their health.

The *Allergen D.A.* identifies your "allergic" response to ten toxins: Bacteria, Antibiotics, Cain, Quinoline or Kaba mixtures; Epoxy, Potassium Dichromate, Animal Hair, Paints, UV Rays, Formaldehyde, Lanolin Alcohol and Chloride (see Your Toxins Identified video on www.biofeedbackbook.com). Most of these categories point to common toxin sources, while others, are less obvious sources. For example, Cain and Kaba mixtures used in anesthetics, cause histamine release which raises the body's inflammation rate. Epoxy and Quinoline are used in adhesives, surface coating and paints. Potassium dichromate is common in cement and other variety of chemicals. Formaldehyde exists in a variety of building material and plastic industries. Lanolin alcohol is often included in ointments, creams, skin care and soap products. Chloride, which is often confused with chlorine, is used in gold-plated items and in costume jewelry.

The second group of panels assesses your body's "coping" level by measuring two key indicators of toxic load. The *Basic Physical Quality D.A.* points to major ways in which you can help your body keep toxicity levels at bay. One measure is hypoxia or proper oxygenation of the cells. Another measure is hydration through water and maintaining a pH level of 3.6 alkalinity. It is crucial to remember that any disease thrives only in an acidic medium. Therefore, alkalinity is ideal in order to prevent disease from occurring.

The *Skin D.A.* is a vital indicator of the body's present state of toxicity levels. The Skin Free Radical Index and Skin Immunity Index are two indicators. Their relationship is key to understanding how toxins impact your immunity. The skin is your largest organ and, as such, is the largest area of exposure to toxins. Here you can appreciate the fact that this subcategory of Skin Free Radical Index, measured through your skin molecules, assesses the degree to which these toxins are prevalent just under your skin. These free radicals have the potential to damage your DNA, your body's proteins and cause cancers (Chapter 3). The Skin Immunity Index evaluates the "health state" of your skin faced with toxins it cannot remove. Your personal value measurement of the first panel is in an inverse relationship to the second one. In other words, the higher your free radical value, the lower your skin immunity index.

The liver is the largest detoxifying organ in your body. Its health and function are primordial for reducing your toxic load. The *Liver Function D.A.* measures five liver markers specific to the liver's health. The Detoxification Function is one marker of the liver's capacity to decompose hazardous substances such as alcohol and ammonia, produced through digestion, into harmless substances such as urea, water and carbon dioxide to be excreted out of the body. Should your liver fare poorly in its detoxification function index, it is an indication that your liver is over taxed, possibly, by any of the above or other toxins. This would be a good time to intervene and reduce the liver's work load.

CHAPTER 3
HOW FREE RADICALS AND INFLAMMATION ARE HURTING YOU!

The previous chapter on toxicity elaborated on the types of toxins you are exposed to. This chapter focuses on the effects of toxins overload on the body causing *oxidative stress*, specifically the excess of free radical activity and its impact on your health. The first line of defense, as briefly discussed in Chapter 2, is identifying your toxins and their load in your body. This chapter introduces two more recommendations to help fight back:

1) Improve your nutritional balance (see video Fight Back with Optimized Levels of Nutrients in www.biofeedback book.com)

2) Inhibit and detoxify toxins always (see video Anti-Oxidants & Detoxifiers in www.biofeedbook.com)

Both steps are made possible with the aid of your bio-scan.

The key term above is toxin *overload* caused by excessive amount of free radicals in comparison to your *antioxidant* level. Even though free radicals are normally present in our bodies in small numbers, helping the immune system destroy viruses and bacteria, their overload essentially leads to disease.

What is a free radical? A free radical is an atom or a molecule with one electron. Since electrons need to be paired for a stable chemical structure to occur, the single electron will pair with any other electron from a surrounding molecule. This action then damages that molecule which will, in turn, grab another electron from somewhere else. This chain reaction leaves our cells less robust, prone to disease and aging more quickly than healthy cells. Worse, if free radical electrons steal an electron from your genetic structure or DNA, gene mutation, can occur causing cancer or disease.

How can free radical overload damage your health? Free radicals inhibit special proteins in the brain and cause Alzheimer's disease. They damage blood vessels which can cause (elevated) blood pressure. Equally damaging is their impact on your detoxification system. Free radicals displace good oils in the mitochondrial membrane (refer to Chapter 4), the energy furnace of the cell located inside the cell, and make it impossible to lose weight. They also lower the DHA, a fatty acid necessary for brain and heart health.

Normally, our body maintains a delicate balance between free radicals and anti-oxidants which act like a sponge to sop up free radicals. However, since free radicals are a natural result of metabolism, food digestion and breathing, any other toxins added to our body will overtax it. While, normally, our body maintains an equilibrium between free radicals and antioxidants, this balance is a very delicate one to sustain. So, while you cannot eliminate all free radical activity in your body, reducing the total load of toxin exposure is very beneficial.

How can you detect and measure your toxic load before you experience symptoms of toxicity? The bio-scan will guide you. It not only identifies and measures your toxicity level toward various toxins but the bio-scan will also provide a *comprehensive reading* of your free radical activity under *Skin D.A.* (see Chapter 2). In other words, you will be given a level of "intensity" of your body's response to various toxins measured during your scan. Armed with this information, you can further improve your fight against oxidants by enhancing your own body's defenses: nutrition and anti-oxidants capacity. Address your identified nutritional deficiency by using the *Trace Element D.A.* and *Amino Acid D.A.* panels. Fight with powerful anti-oxidants listed in the *Coenzyme D.A.*

The first recommendation is to enhance your body's own natural detoxification mechanism. For this mechanism to work efficiently you need to optimize your body's nutritional levels of vitamins, minerals and amino acids. If your body is deficient in these areas your body is not in a position to fight back.

Ten vitamins and five minerals levels are measured individually in the *Trace Element D.A.* This panel precisely measures your levels of the minerals (calcium, iron, zinc and selenium) and of the vitamins (A, C, E, K, B1, B2, Folic Acid, B3, B6, B12 and D3) (view Trace Element video on www.biofeedbackbook.com). Although this is not a comprehensive list of all vitamins and minerals, those listed here have a significant impact on your detoxification efficacy. Being aware of the need to supplement with multivitamins and minerals is important. Being cognizant of your specific body levels and monitoring them in a follow-up bio-scan can be achieved very easily. For example, one of calcium's primordial functions in your body is to protect bones and teeth from lead by inhibiting its absorption. A deficiency in calcium leads to lead absorption which is then deposited in teeth and bones. Excessive amounts of iron can lead to the production of free radicals. Another vital anti-oxidant, largely neglected, is selenium. One of its principal functions is to protect the immune system by preventing the formation of free radicals. The same is true for zinc.

All vitamins are necessary. Vitamins A, C and E are very powerful antioxidants and in turn extremely important. Vitamin A, for example, reduces the oxidation (or toxicity) of your DNA. Vitamin C is an electron donor. It also aids *glutathione* (measured under *Coenzyme D.A.*) to bind with chemicals thus facilitating the pulling of chemicals out of the bloodstream (refer to Chapters 4, 6 & 7). As for glutathione, it can grab onto hundreds of types of environmental chemicals (toxins) and drag them right out of the bloodstream into the liver, then to the gallbladder to finally be flushed down through the intestine and excreted from the body (see Chapter 5). A marvellous system altogether provided, of course, you are not constipated.

During constipation, the glutathione falls off the toxin chemical and the chemical is reabsorbed into the body. Gastrointestinal health is, therefore, a necessity in detoxification (see Chapter 5).

High vitamin C levels cause elevation of the killer cells in over 70% of people. It is the first line of defense needed to fight off infection as well as cancer cells. Since your body cannot manufacture vitamin C, it is essential to supplement it through food or in the form of supplements.Vitamins C and E work synergistically as antioxidants.

Minerals sustain life. Every living cell on this planet depends on minerals for proper function and structure. Minerals are needed for the proper composition of body fluids, the formation of blood and bone, the maintenance of healthy nerve function and the regulation of muscle tone, including that of the muscles of the cardiovascular system. Like vitamins, minerals function as helpers, enabling the body to perform its functions, including energy production, growth and healing. Minerals are stored primarily in the body's bone and muscle tissue.

The *Trace Element D.A.* panel measures the following minerals: calcium, iron, selenium and zinc. Calcium, a bulk mineral, is needed in larger amounts than trace minerals. However both groups are needed. Calcium is not merely needed for bone, teeth and gum health (see Chapter 5), but is also vital for the maintenance of a regular heartbeat and in the transmission of nerve pulses. It lowers cholesterol and helps prevent cardiovascular disease. Many, many more essential health measures depend on calcium. It is important to know that our body does not produce calcium. You need to supplement your body with calcium supplements. Clarification on the process of calcium absorption can be found in Chapter 5. However, it is important to note that the amino acid *lysine*, measured in the *Amino Acid D.A.*, is needed for calcium absorption. This is just another "link" example, amongst others, of how the bio-scan can draw attention to the link between your calcium absorption level and your lysine level.

The mineral iron is found in the largest amount in the blood. Its most important function is the production of hemoglobin and the oxygenation of red blood cells. While it is common to link iron deficiency with anemia, it is also possible for iron deficiency to be due to vitamin B6 or B12 deficiency. These two vitamins can be the underlying cause of anemia. They are measured under the *Trace Element D.A.* It is also well to remember that excessive iron intake, as mentioned earlier, can cause problems which lead to the production of free radicals, heart disease and cancer.

Selenium's principal function is to inhibit the oxidation of lipids (fats) as a component of the enzyme glutathione (refer to Chapter 5). It is a vital antioxidant especially when it is combined with vitamin E. It protects the immune system by preventing the formation of free radicals. It plays a vital role in regulating the effects of thyroid hormone.

Zinc is important in prostate gland function and the growth of the reproductive organs. This function can be cross checked in the *Prostate Function D.A.* measuring your prostate health (refer to Chapter 6). It is required for protein synthesis, promotes healthy immune and the healing of wounds. It also enhances the acuity of taste and smell.

Equally essential are your body's amino acids levels. The *Amino Acid D.A.* measures the ten essential amino acids you require (consult Amino Acid video on www.biofeedback book.com). There are approximately twenty-eight commonly known amino acids that are combined in various ways to create the hundreds of different types of proteins your body needs. The liver produces about 80% of amino acids while your diet must supplement the remaining 20%. The amino acids measured under the above panel are referred to as *essential* amino acids.

Why amino acids? They are the building blocks of protein in your body (see Chapter 4). While, most people supplement with vitamins and some minerals, few people are aware of the vital role amino acids play. They play an important role   in allowing vitamins and minerals to be effective. Amongst the ten essential amino acids measured in your *Amino Acid D.A.* we already referred to the importance of lysine with respect to calcium absorption. As well, lysine aids in the production of antibodies, hormones, enzymes, collagen, tissue repair, muscle protein as well as fight cold sores and herpes. Tryptophan is necessary for normal sleep duration (refer to Chapter 6). Methionine breaks down fats to prevent build-up in the liver and arteries. Leucine protects your muscles and acts as fuel for them. It lowers elevated blood sugar and aids in increasing your human growth hormones. Threonine is good for your heart, central nervous system, prevents fatty liver build-up, enhances your immune system and will help with some types of depression. So whether you are concerned about your blood sugar, fatty liver, sleep inadequacy, or feeling a bit depressed or moody, checking your amino acids with a bio scan can help optimize the levels. Only a balanced pool of amino acids can balance your metabolism to keep you healthy.

The second recommendation, to fight back against free radicals, is understanding how to utilize antioxidants and detoxifiers. Unlike some common perception, the two substances are not synonymous even though they both work to detoxify the body.

Antioxidants are substances that block or inhibit free radical damage. Specific vitamins, minerals and enzymes help prevent cancer and other disorders by protecting cells against damage from oxidation. Vitamins A, C and E and the mineral selenium are some of the antioxidants measured in your bio-scan and discussed in chapter 2. The coenzyme CoQ10 is another antioxidant measured. It is a well researched, medically proven antioxidant, hailed for its multiple benefits. The greatest concentration of CoQ10 is found in the heart, followed by the liver, kidney, spleen and pancreas. It is essential for cell health, therefore, as you will read in chapter 4, it is basic to your state of health. Its presence in the mitochondria (the cells' energy production centers) is very indicative of its primordial role (refer to Chapter 4). This coenzyme is measured in the *Coenzyme D.A.* and would be useful if replenished consistently (see video Coenzymes in www.biofeedbackbook.com). It is important to note that your body uses up an antioxidant molecule forever with every molecule of chemical that is detoxified. Therefore, you need to constantly replenish that supply on a daily basis (refer to Chapters 4 & 7).

Detoxifiers are substances that reduce the buildup of free radical activity in the body. Among the most versatile detoxifiers produced by the body is glutathione measured as well in the *Coenzyme D.A.* Here is why: glutathione is both an antioxidant and a detoxifier. Glutathione is a protein produced in the liver from three amino acids. This substance is a powerful antioxidant, protecting against cellular damage. The largest stores of glutathione are found in the liver, where it detoxifies harmful compounds so that they can be excreted through the bile. Some glutathione is released from the liver and directly into the bloodstream, where it helps maintain the integrity of red blood cells and protect white blood cells. Glutathione is also found in the lungs and the intestinal tract where it is needed for carbohydrates metabolism and the breakdown of oxidized fats. It is also a powerful detoxifier of heavy metals and drugs. It metabolizes oxygen molecules before they can harm the cells. When you monitor your glutathione level in your bio-scan, you will have an added bonus. The rate at which you age directly correlates with reduced concentrations of glutathione in the cellular fluids. As we grow older, it is worthwhile to keep this valuable antioxidant / detoxifier well stocked in your body. Feel better, look younger, at whatever age, is a win-win strategy!

CHAPTER 4
BODY HEALTH COMES FROM CELL HEALTH

Chapters 1, 2 and 3 gave you an overview of how your bio-scan provides you with specific personal data you can use to identify and address any deficiency, imbalance or health related issues, thereby optimizing your wellness. Chapter 4 takes a closer look at the *WHAT, WHERE* and *HOW* everything is about ENERGY! How do we define energy? Where is it made? How to nourish it instead of deplete it? These are some questions that guide this chapter.

The entire human body is made of cells, each of which contains its own genetic material or DNA - a long string of molecules that tell the cell what to do. In a healthy body, cells divide at a controlled rate so as to grow and repair damaged tissue and replace dying cells. You may remember this is the technology employed in the bio-scan. This predetermined rate of cell division is mostly controlled by what is known as the mitochondria which keeps our body energized and healthy. In the previous chapter you read that oxidative stress threatens your daily performance, your quality of life and how anti-oxidants/detoxifiers are your best line of defence. These systems are created within and by the mitochondria!! For the purposes of this chapter we shall focus on how to maintain mitochondrial health.

There are over ten million billion *mitochondria* in the human body. Each cell contains an average of 300-400 of these magnificent nourishing signaling centers. They are composed of tiny packages of enzymes that turn nutrients into cellular energy. They create 90% of cellular energy necessary to sustain life and growth. They are considered the "powerhouse of the cell". Basically they are responsible for producing cell energy, and by extension, your body's energy. They are responsible for generating cellular energy through a process called ATP or Adenosine Tri-phosphate (immediate source of cell energy). This is your energy supply summed up in those three letters - your ATP - and it is produced directly by your mitochondrial system. Mitochondrial failure causes cell injury leading to cell death. When multiple organ cells die there is organ failure. Basically, the above answers WHAT energy is and WHERE it is generated.

HOW does the mitochondria ensure your cell health and by extension your body health? Cells do not survive on their own. Their health or dysfunction depends almost entirely on the mitochondria. Mitochondria are *metabolic signaling centers* that influence an organism's physiology by regulating communication between cells and tissues. They are like the "traffic signals", ensuring traffic safety. Through the mitochondria control of cell growth and death rate, we can easily see how crucial "cell activity signaling" would be in leading either to healthy cells, abnormal or possibly cancerous cells. Most of the time our bodies have the ability to destroy these abnormal cells and maintain a sort of cellular equilibrium. However, if a crucial portion of the DNA is destroyed (by free radical activity), the abnormal cells can no longer be controlled. Obviously, we need to protect the cell process at all cost.

Interestingly, the mitochondria have their own DNA structure (mtDNA) which guides their signaling system which is different from our cells' DNA system. So we have two DNA systems, each one independent in its structure yet interdependent on the other. Both need to stay well-functioning in order for your ATP supply to continue nourishing you by keeping a balanced cell activity and giving you energy. Of course this is a very simplified way to present these complex systems. Many fascinating articles on the internet address mitochondria history, functions and dysfunctions. They are implicated in common diseases like diabetes, metabolic syndrome, cancer, obesity and cardiovascular health. As well, mitochondria dysfunction has been associated with new era diseases such Fibromyalgia, Chronic Fatigue Syndrome and Lupus, amongst others.

The underlying support system of any cell comes down to its mitochondrial support function. The bio-scan measures two vital components of mitochondrial health: calcium in *Trace Element D.A.* and coenzyme Q10 in *Coenzyme D.A.* (see video on Calcium and Coenzyme Q10 for Cell Health www.biofeed backbook.com). It is important to recognize that the function calcium performs goes far beyond the bone mineral density concern. One of the mitochondria's crucial functions is to help preserve the cell's environment. This specifically involves calcium which is a "signaling molecule" alerting the cell to respond to the body's processes or needs. This *calcium is stored in and is regulated by the mitochondria.* The mitochondria determines when and how much calcium to release to the cell for its necessary activities. Should the mitochondria dispense calcium unnecessarily to the cell it would be detrimental to the finely tuned regulation of processes within the cell. Even cancers are associated with defect in the mitochondrial signaling between it and the cell's nucleus. Clearly, mutations in the mitochondrial DNA, or mtDNA, play a role in tumor metastasis where the signaling of cell multiplication becomes defective. Interestingly, even diabetics or pre-diabetics now show a very consistent decline in mitochondrial function. So it is crucial to keep your calcium levels healthy and use your bio-scan to measure those levels readily in the *Trace Element D.A.*

Another way to protect your mitochondria against possible mutations of its DNA (different from your cell's DNA) is to keep your coenzyme Q10 levels optimized. In order to truly appreciate this enzyme function, consider this: even with the presence of sufficient amounts of vitamins, minerals, water and other nutrients, without enzymes, life as we know it could not exist. Why? Enzymes are catalysts. Catalysts promote, encourage, spark a biochemical reaction in the body. Now it is easier to see how enzymes, the "sparks of life" precipitate, speed up, the hundreds of thousands of biochemical reactions in the body that control life's processes. They assist in practically all bodily functions, detoxification being one of the most life-saving processes. There are two groups of enzymes: digestive enzymes (breaking down the food for energy) and metabolic ones. The latter catalyzes the various chemical reactions within the cells promoting energy production and detoxification.

Coenzyme Q10 is a metabolic enzyme as well as a powerful antioxidant (see Chapter 3). This substance plays a critical role in the production of energy in every cell of the body. Coenzyme Q10 is present in the mitochondria of all the cells in the body. It is vital because it carries into the cells the energy-laden protons and electrons that are used to produce your ATP, the immediate source of cellular energy. This is a constant process because the body can store only a small quantity of ATP at any one time. It is believed that as many as 75% of people, over fifty, may be deficient in coenzyme Q10. Deficiency can lead to cardiovascular disease. Within the mitochondria-- the cells' energy production centers-- coenzyme Q10 helps to metabolize the fats and carbohydrates. It also helps to maintain the flexibility of cell membranes. The heart muscle, followed by the liver, kidney, spleen and pancreas, have the highest level of CoQ10 of any organ. Without enough CoQ10 the heart cannot circulate the blood effectively. This is another good reason to measure and monitor your CoQ10 enzyme in your bio-scan.

Another *signaling molecule* for all your cells is Nitric Oxide. This dynamic molecule is a key signaling molecule throughout your body. It is produced by the endothelial (inner) cells lining the arteries and acts as a potent vaso-dialator that relaxes the arteries. Therefore, nitric oxide plays a role in blood pressure and overall circulation (see Chapters 1 & 2). It also curbs inflammation and oxidative stress (see Chapter 3). This essential compound is generated in the brain and involved in neurotransmission. Nitric oxide's benefits also include protection against dementia and other neurodegenerative disorders. In the gastrointestinal tract, it helps to regulate intestinal peristalsis and the secretion of mucus and gastric acid (refer to Chapter 5). It is also involved in insulin signaling monitored in the (*Blood Lipids D.A.* and *Pancreatic Function D.A.*); bone remodeling (*Rheumatoid Bone Disease D.A.*); respiratory function (*Lung Function D.A.*) and mitochondrial creation and utilization of cellular energy ATP function.

How do you optimize your nitric oxide levels? Even though the bio-scan does not measure specifically for nitric oxide levels, it guides you to protect its production since nitric oxide is synthesized from the amino acid arginine as well as two other amino acids. Therefore, it is important to monitor your arginine level in the *Amino Acid D.A.* panel of your bio scan. Two other components necessary for your nitric oxide levels are physical exercise and consuming foods rich in dietary nitrates. Equally important is to supplement with antioxidants because they protect the endothelium (inner membrane of the arteries supplying blood to all tissues) and guard against nitric oxide degradation. Ensure that you are supplementing daily with an antioxidant rich with multivitamins and minerals (refer to Chapter 7). These supplements will go a long way to help protect your mitochondria for life.

CHAPTER 5
GUT HEALTH: THE ENGINE BEHIND THE BODY

The gastrointestinal tract consists of the stomach, the small and large intestines. It is the powerhouse behind all the nutrition we need in order to function and survive. Although every cell in the body has a detoxification plant right inside of it, i.e. the mitochondria, over half of the detoxification for the entire body occurs in the gut.

The intestinal lining houses half of the immune system for the whole body, as well as, half of the detoxification system. Because of this, you can not completely heal any disease, regardless of its label, until the gut is healthy. Unfortunately, most people's intestines are loaded with nasty bacteria (usually from eating out frequently or from processed foods) and with yeasts, like Candida (from antibiotics, birth control pills or a diet high in sweets).

However, once you understand your digestive mechanism, you will be in a better position to help your gut. There are two digestive processes involved: the mechanical and the chemical. Whereas, the mouth and stomach take care of the mechanical digestion i.e., the breaking down, chewing and ingesting of food, the small intestine is where the chemical digestion takes place. It is where 90% of the digestion and absorption of food occurs, whereas, the other 10% take place in the stomach and large intestine. Therefore the main function of the small intestine is the absorption of nutrients and minerals from food. It uses enzymes like bile (stored in the gallbladder) to break down material into a form that can then be absorbed and assimilated into the tissues of the body. The large intestine is responsible for storing and eliminating waste material within 24 hours in order to prevent toxin re-absorption by the body.

Chemical digestion breaks down proteins, lipids (fats) and carbohydrates. Once broken down they are absorbed by the gastrointestinal tract cells into the bloodstream. In fact, water, electrolytes (like sodium, chloride, iodine, iron, calcium, vitamin D, magnesium, potassium), and all vitamins and minerals are absorbed through the small intestine's chemical digestion.

So why is your GI tract essential to your health? Imagine what your healthy GI tract does for you. Not only does it provide good absorption of nutrients, proper elimination of waste but it also maintains a healthy flora where the good and bad bacteria, entering your GI through food, are balanced. In addition the GI tract releases hormones from your bile and saliva enzymes to help regulate the digestive process.

How can you attain and maintain a healthy GI? The bio-scan will guide you every step of the way. The *Gastrointestinal Function D.A.* and the *Large Intestine Function D.A.* panels reflect the health state of the stomach, small and large intestine as well as the colon. Without a healthy GI tract you can neither metabolize nor absorb nutrients.

Nutrients, their metabolism and absorption are essential to keeping your body healthy in order to fight back. For example, metabolism, as in glucose metabolism, is a chemical trans-formation where insulin promotes the liver to utilize glucose and convert it to a metabolised form of sugar. In contrast, absorption refers to the uptake of these metabolized sugars as nutrient through the wall of the intestine before they enter the bloodstream. Both systems work in tandem and must work effectively to deliver nutrients to the body.

How do you optimize your nutrient absorption? The first step is to identify any GI issues you may have by referring to your bio-scan on *Gastrointestinal Function D.A.* and on the *Large Intestine Function D.A.* panels. Both panels measure specifically the peristalsis (the contraction and relaxation movement) and the absorption in the stomach and in both intestines for further nutrients processing.

The first measurement is that of the peristalsis (refer to Gastrointestinal Function Panel in www.biofeedbackbook.com). The Gastric Peristalsis Function Coefficient, the Small Intestine Peristalsis, and the Large Intestine Peristalsis Function measure each part's peristalsis movement respectively. The peristalsis movement in the stomach grinds the food into a paste for further processing. As it enters the small intestine, this paste is further liquefied through peristalsis and gastric acids.

The second measurement is that of the gastric absorption by the same gut parts (refer to Gastric Absorption Video in www.biofeedbackbook.com). Absorption depends on the chemical digestion which requires the secretion of gastric juices: hydrochloric acid and pepsin. For example, pepsin is secreted by the stomach's gastric gland and is measured under Pepsin Secretion Coefficient. This measurement is a good indicator of the level of gastric juices secretion in the stomach. A level of pepsin lower than the normal range is indicative of a digestive absorption issue. The same chemical process takes place in the small intestine and is measured in the Small Intestine Absorption Function Coefficient. It is a crucial indicator of your nutrient absorption levels. Here is where sugars, protein and fat are absorbed. This function underlines your nutritional health as the sugar is decomposed into simple sugar; the proteins are converted into amino acids and fat into fatty acid etc. The small intestine is also where the absorption of water occurs.

The third measurement refers to colon's health. Bacterial level and any fermentation caused by a "lazy" colon are measured by the Intestinal Bacteria Coefficient and by the Intraluminal Pressure Coefficient respectively (consult video on Large Intestine in www.biofeedbackbook.com). Should your large intestine prove to be "lazy" in the peristalsis movement there will be intestinal flatulence (gas, bloating, abdominal distension) measured on the same panel. These symptoms are not simply "socially awkward inconveniences", rather, they are symptoms of unhealthy gut. Rather than ignoring these common symptoms, you may consider reversing them. Their presence may well indicate gut toxicity which can shut down the immune system. For example, the harmful fungus, Candida, releases yeast toxins in the gut and can lead to leaky gut syndrome. Candidiasis thrives in the body if the pH balance is upset. Candidiasis disables the friendly bacteria lactobacilli from metabolizing sugars.

Also, unsuspecting external factors can equally compromise your gut health. For example, exposure to mycotoxins, produced by black mold toxins, destroy the gut lining. High levels of ammonia gas, caused by bad bacteria in the gut, lowers serotonin levels.

All of the above indicators point to the GI tract as a prominent part of the immune system. Your gut health is all connected and is worth protecting.

CHAPTER 6
BIOFEEDBACK SCAN FINDS YOUR WEAKNESSES

So how else can your bio-scan help keep you healthy? Monitoring any health issues by using over thirty different health related panels is a great vehicle especially since you are probably already aware of your health state. Through the scan any "unsuspected", "unnoticeable" conditions will be revealed. This is no reason to be concerned, since almost all conditions are reversible, with awareness, proper protection measures and adequate supplementation.

Here are some examples. More people are aware of the links between mental and physical wellness today. Both are interrelated and interdependent. Yet, it is not likely for a person to be able to identify those links without some clear indication as to their connection in the body, especially at early stages. Consider the brain for example. The *Brain Nerve D.A.* panel offers a guiding hand. Under the entry Sentiment Index, for example, the bio-scan measures your body's response to stress by examining negative emotions which may emanate from negative feelings such as upset, sadness, anxiety and apathy. The link between negative emotions and stress are well documented (watch video on Brain Nerve in biofeedback book.com). Yet stress is often viewed as a psychological problem. More and more evidence supports the fact that elevated stress levels have very real physical effects on heart beat, blood pressure and cause a greater degree of tension in the muscles. Becoming cognizant of this factor during your wellness journey is instrumental in guiding you to consider, and very realistically, optimize both your physical and mental health.

Another vital indicator of elevated stress is *sleep deprivation*. We typically associate stress with work, family responsibilities, financial concerns, time management etc. We often overlook the fact that sleep deficiency causes stress. Sleep deficiency stresses the immune system, and, if it is not addressed, or lasts a long period of time, will disrupt one's daily function and performance. Most people are aware of what Sleep Apnea entails. However, they are unaware of its symptoms and usually may be unaware they suffer from this sleep deprivation condition. The reason is simple. When a person is unaware that insomnia or morning fatigue is due to sleep apnea and not just a bad night sleep, he or she may waste an opportunity to investigate the root cause of their poor sleep. The bio-scan detects Sleep Apnea in the *Obesity Panel D.A.* and many are surprised to find out they indeed suffer from Sleep Apnea and are unaware of its affect on them (refer to video on Obesity Panel in www.biofeedbackbook.com). Sleep Apnea can be addressed once a person is tested in a sleep laboratory and is given corrective oxygenation equipment or device for sleep purposes.

Two other markers of sleep issues are the level of tryptophan, an essential amino acid and the pineal gland secretion. Both are tested in the bio-scan. Tryptophan is used by the brain to produce serotonin, a necessary neurotransmitter that transfers nerve impulses from one cell to another and is responsible for normal sleep. Consequently, tryptophan helps to combat depression, insomnia and to stabilize moods. Another marker for sleep deprivation is the pineal gland secretion level (see Endocrine System video on www.biofeedbackbook.com). It controls the secretion of the sleep hormone melatonin. The gland shrinks in daylight and expands in dark environment when it produces melatonin. By producing this hormone, the gland releases a time signal to the central nervous system which then regulates your circadian (daily) rhythm of sleep and awake time. In short, your sleep duration and timing depend on your circadian cycle. Identifying "unsuspected" sleep concerns is usually a shortcut to determine possible fatigue issues.

Prostate health is essential to a man's physical, emotional and sexual health. The *Prostate D.A.* panel is probably a man's best friend (watch Prostate Health video on www.biofeedbackbook.com). It alerts you to any prostate issue early on, as opposed to detection in the later stages when a PSA test may be needed. Three entries are measured in that panel. The first entry measures the Degree of Prostatic Hyperplasia and refers to the degree to which the prostate volume gradually increases, forming what is called prostatic hyperplasia. The course of *prostatic hyperplasia* develops slowly so there are no symptoms early on. This is one very important reading which does not involve any invasive or formal testing. An aggravated prostatic hyperplasia will cause some degree of urinary bladder obstruction which may alert you to prostate issue. The bio- scan, however, measures the slightest degree of hyperplasia. A reading over the range indicated (1.023-3.230) alerts the person to a developing tendency of hyperplasia.

The second entry measured is the degree of Prostatic Calcification. Fibrosis, a scar left by prostate inflammation, is a precursor for prostate stones or calcification which generally breed bacteria and more complications. Again, the range for healthy prostate is given in numerical value in order to help you identify any "abnormality". Thus, the scan can determine any degree of inflammation of the prostate.

The third entry measures the Prostatitis Syndrome level in a person. Since prostatitis can be asymptomatic at first, early identification is important as Prostatitis Syndrome is reversible in early stages. Once you are alerted to this possibility you can address it more quickly, thereby increasing the chances of reversal, while you monitor it in a follow-up scan.

Prostate health is a vital component of a male's sexual and reproductive health, as well, as being an indicator of overall health. The point here is that early detection, through a one minute bio-scan, is a worthwhile investment of your time. A non-invasive bio scan detects the health of your prostate while you wait.

Similarly, the *Gynecology D.A.* panel can be a woman's guide to her reproductive organs and sexual health. For example, the panel measures the female hormone production needed for sexual and reproductive health. Progesterone is amongst the hormones measured (see video on Gynecology Health in www.biofeedbackbook.com). The panel also measures some "undetectable" but important markers for a woman's health. Three markers are: vaginitis, cervicitis and ovarian cysts. Mostly, unnoticed and undetected at first, these conditions are reversible when attended to early on. Of course, close monitoring of the degree of development is always recommended. For example, the Vaginitis Coefficient refers to a kind of inflammation of the vagina and is a common condition for some women. It occurs when the natural defence function of the vagina breaks down and pathogens (microbes, bacteria... etc.) intrude easily and cause inflammation. Young girls and postmenopausal women are more liable to infection. The vaginitis coefficient is measured by the bio-scan and will point to any mild or moderate, as well, as severe vaginitis issue.

Equally important for women is hormonal production. For most women, hormone production begins to slow down when they reach their thirties and continues to diminish as they age. Many years before a woman stops ovulating, her ovaries slow their production of the hormones estrogen, progesterone and testosterone. Progesterone, for example, works as a counterpart to estrogen. Beyond the reproductive function of progesterone, this hormone has a calming effect on the brain and appears to affect other aspects of the central nervous system's function. Since hormones are the "chemical messengers" to all body organs to stimulate growth, healing and reproduction, understanding and monitoring your hormone levels, whether you are female or male, at whatever age, is an integral part of health and wellness. Like all organs, the glands need nutritional support, especially when stress depletes the body's stores of nutrients. A quick measurement of your hormonal level will save you guessing why you feel fatigued, sleepy, moody, brain fogged, stressed, always hungry or lacking sexual drive.

CHAPTER 7
THE THREE STEPS TO HEALTH

Two defence measures will help you reach your optimum health and maintain a sense of wellness. The first defence measure is to empower yourself with knowledge about your body. Let "your body speak to you" through your first biofeedback and sequential bio-scans, *YOUR WELLNESS GPS!* guide. Your bio-scan results are emailed to you the same day in a compositive scan, which indicate all your "actual measurements" in all scanned categories. Reading your scan results on your own is made simply by comparing your Actual Measurement Value to the Normal Range value in any one given entry (refer to the video on Measurements in www.biofeedbackbook.com) . Nothing is simpler. You will be able to keep this first bio-scan record and compare it to your follow-up bio-scans in order to establish, for yourself, the degree of improvement in each entry. It is all in black and white.

Equally, you will benefit from the "underestimated" advantage of testing your whole body as a UNIT, a dynamic system, where all readings connect to your overall sense of being. Over thirty panels will reveal to you the "what", the "where" and the "why" certain sub-health issues need your attention. Should you be on prescription drugs, or under the care of your medical doctor for any particular condition, you will be comforted to know that your scan data can guide you very closely in monitoring your particular health concern. Re-scanning every three months or less can empower you with the knowledge of your body's ability and guide you to optimized health. You can do all that in real time at the same time!

The second measure is, armed with the insight, you are more equipped to fight back by optimizing your health. Today we battle disease by means of drugs, surgery, radiation and other therapies but, true health can be attained only by maintaining a healthy, properly functioning immune system. Weakening the immune system, results in increased susceptibility to every type of illness.

To fight back you need to follow *three steps:*

1) Reduce your toxic load
2) Guard your Immune with your life
3) Nourish your body

The first step is to reduce your toxic load. Many poisons surround us so do your part. The first poison you need to avoid as much as possible is sugar- in all its forms- fructose, glucose, lactose and sucrose. There is no other description for it, sugar is poison. Sugar is poisoning you and it comes in hidden measures and products you consume even when you think you have read the label. Check again and somewhere you will find a form of syrup, molasses, dextrose...etc. Check your fruit intake and try to follow the *Glycemic Index* (sugar level) of the fruits you consume, especially tropical ones, which are high in fructose.

The second poison is plastic. Reduce all your plastics including your water bottles. Use glass bottles and mix in them your alkaline water. That is a good start. Replace as many plastic containers / bottles in your home or refrigerator with glass containers. They are breakable and heavier but, based on the knowledge of phthalates (plastic off-gas from plastic products), you can rest assured your body will appreciate your effort.

Detoxify your home. If you can, replace your household toxic products with natural, eco-friendly ones. Read the label and eliminate: chlorine, ammonia and formaldehyde. Avoid phosphates, parabens, triclosan and phthalates. Try products that use herbs like thyme and citric acid to clean. Wash away dirt with glycerine, aloe and vitamin E. At all times avoid DEET. Instead, look for products that substitute essential oils, like peppermint, cinnamon, lemongrass, thyme and geranium, for mouthwash and toothpaste. Rely on lavender oil as an effective insect repellent and mold detoxifier. From shampoo and deodorant, to furniture polish and laundry detergent, convert them all into natural products.

Replacing your carpets with hardwood flooring would be a great asset. Test your home for mold and radon gas by checking for leaks from the ground into your basement. Always air out your house, or office, daily, if possible. Fresh air is a direct way to remove mycotoxins from your immediate environment.

Detoxify your body. Use infra red sauna for twenty minutes once or twice a week. The infra red rays draw out, through sweat, the toxins deposited under the epidermis layer of your skin. If you feel adventurous, but serious about your gut health, a coffee enema is very effective in releasing toxic waste deposited in the colon. It will remove waste toxins accumulating and fermenting in the gut. Use organic enema coffee available online. Treat yourself to an *Ionics* foot bath treatment once a month. Heavy metals, such as lead and iron, measured by the bio-scan, are released before your eyes as you watch the water change into different colors. You will see brown, blue and aquamarine patches released through the ionization process removing mercury and lead from your kidneys and liver.

Give your family and yourself the gift of charcoal shower filter available online to reduce some of the more than one thousand toxic chemicals in our water supply. Be weary of MSG used as flavouring ingredient in restaurants. It raises the levels of glutamate (an excitatory chemical) in the brain which, in turn, elevates brain toxicity. Reduce pesticide levels in your food supply whenever possible. Fruits and vegetables should be soaked in water and vinegar for 15 minutes, in order to remove as many pesticides as possible, even if they are organic products.

De-stress yourself however you can and follow the right regimen of some daily physical activity. Consume healthy foods and always keep your social life "active". Always remember to get your deep sleep nightly. This is equally vital for defending your body. Monitor your sleep habits and improve upon them. Follow up on your bio-scan and watch for your level of tryptophan. Do not settle for restless nights as a matter of habit. It is like living life sporadically, that is, when you are not feeling so fatigued. Your energy level will be the first symptom to watch for.

The second step is to guard your immune with your life! Monitor its performance in the *Immune System D.A.* (watch the video on Immune System in www.biofeedbackbook.com). Your bio-scan will confirm your levels of hydration and oxygenation. Start with good hydration and oxygenation as suggested by your bio-scan in the *Basic Physical Quality D.A.* (consult the video on Basic Physical Quality in www.biofeedbackbook.com). Hydrate with alkaline water to balance your pH level and flush out your toxins. Water is the only liquid that can do that. Add two to three drops of lemon per glass to make your water alkaline. Your bio-scan will confirm your proper levels. Oxygenation is giving life to your cells. Deep "belly" breathing is the only way to get oxygen to all body cells including your brain cells.

Monitor your endocrine system of glands and their secretion. They secrete hormones into the bloodstream. The endocrine is considered to be the largest system in the body.

This is so because the hormones, released by various glands, send messages to the central nervous system to perform a certain task. For instance, the hormone melatonin secreted by the pineal gland, instructs the central nervous system to slow down your body activities in order for you to fall asleep. In fact, the endocrine and the central nervous system are considered to be the two largest systems in the body. So monitoring your endocrine activity, will serve you well.

The *Endocrine System D.A.* will assist you well (see Endocrine System video in www.biofeedbackbook.com). It measures the pituitary, thyroid, parathyroid, thymus, pineal and adrenal glands. The pituitary gland is considered the most important human gland. It secretes hormones such as the human growth hormone and thyroid stimulating hormone. Consider the Thyroid Gland and its close connection to the central nervous system. Both the Thyroid and the central nervous system are referred to as the two major biological information systems in the body. The Thyroid releases thyroid hormones once it is stimulated by the nervous system to do so. Those hormones are sent to the corresponding organ and produce a physiological effect. The Parathyroid Hormone Secretion Index measures your parathyroid secretion. It affects the metabolism of calcium, regulates its concentration and function. The thymus gland secretes thymosin, a hormone that is critical to proper immune system function. The adrenal gland secretes stress hormones which can increase blood pressure, heart rate and elevate blood glucose. The pineal gland regulates your sleep cycle. Briefly, the endocrine system is integral to body functions.

The third step is to nourish your body with the right supplements, thereby enabling your immune system to do its job. You now posses a means, a tool, your bio-scan which will help you measure your starting level and your optimized level of nutrition. Monitor the levels. From multivitamins, minerals, blood sugar, bone mineral health, gut health, brain function to endocrine performance and more, your follow-up bio-scan is a personal record of your progress.

So why should you supplement your body,especially if you are a young person? In the Journal of the American Medical Association (2002) doctors recommended that every adult regardless of age, health needs or gender, take a daily multivitamin to fill the nutritional gaps in his or her diet. If optimizing your health and wellness is your goal, then you should consider only quality supplements. Pharmacopia is the ancient natural science based on the health benefits and curing capacity of plants, herbs, spices and their oils. It is the science behind pharmacology. Today it is in your interest to bring back the "natural" science into your everyday life.

Your bio-scan visit includes supplement recommendations for your specific health concern or condition. Your consultation with the therapist, after your bio-scan, is essentially devoted to determining your health needs and providing you with vital nutritional guidance. This will make your follow-up bio-scan an invaluable experience.

Even though, natural supplements should not interfere with prescription drugs, it is always advisable to check with your doctor when considering additional supplements.

Nutrition is all about the supplement *absorption level* as mentioned earlier. Most off-the-shelf supplements have 5-10% absorption level. You waste your money and the opportunity to address a nutritional deficiency. Worse, some mal-absorbed supplements may cause more harm as they are not absorbed and are then "deposited" somewhere in the body. Calcification, due to mal-absorbed calcium stored in the body, is one example of mal absorption catching the medical community by surprise.

The right strength and choice of ingredients is tantamount to the supplement's efficacy. Save the guess work as to how many milligrams of this, that or the other nutrient, you should combine. Leave that to the experts while you benefit from their research.

Absorption of natural products is highly effective but takes longer to reach its full effect. Typical multivitamins present two main problems: low mineral solubility (absorption) and excess free radical generation in your body. Scientifically formulated natural supplements avoid these issues. By binding minerals, similarly to the way they are bound in nature, these minerals are more available for absorption in your body. Taking effective supplements, which are 95% absorbed, patented, medically proven, published in medical journals and reasonably priced, is a very wise decision.

Vitamin and mineral supplements do not cover a comprehensive list of nutrients. Other nutrients should be included in your supplements. For example, daily Omega 3's is primordial for brain, eye, heart, joints, and total health needs. Your Omega 3's need to provide at least 1000 mg DHA/EPA per serving for multiple health benefits to occur. There is cardi-Omega EPA specifically for heart health and Coldwater Omega 3's for the total body needs. Coldwater Omega is especially formulated to be absorbed with water since it is, essentially, fish oils which do not mix with water. You will be hard pressed to find that information on an Omega bottle.

Grapeseed extract for heart health, saw palmetto, berry, and pumpkin seed for the prostate; blueberry, bilberry for eyesight; and twelve grams of fiber daily for your gut health are necessary nutrients for complete health. These ingredients have shown to be effective in multiple clinical studies.

For your bone health do not just take calcium. Supplement it with K2-D3 (potassium and vitamin D3) to effectively metabolise this complicated but necessary mineral. For your bone, teeth and, definitely, your mitochondrial health, calcium absorption is a must. K2-D3 (potassium and vitamin D) is the ideal nutrient. As you know D3 is necessary for calcium absorption but recently scientists indicated that along with D3, K2 is needed for calcium to be attached to your bones and teeth. Unquestionably, D3 is essential to the creation of the hormone calcitrol which is required for proper absorption of calcium. But once calcium is in the blood, it needs to be attached to the bones, if not, it can remain in the bloodstream where it may deposit in other parts of the body. This is where vitamin K2 is essential to activate the proteins that move the calcium from the bloodstream to your bones. Without K2 the proteins cannot be activated and it is difficult to redirect the calcium.

Your CoQ10 is essential for antioxidant support. It is an essential nutrient for energy creation, supporting a healthy heart, nerve and immune function (refer to Chapter 6).

Nitric Oxide (referred to in Chapter 4) is the new miracle discovery. Increase your level of Nitric Oxide and live longer and healthier! Dubbed by Canadian media as the "Miracle Molecule", nitric oxide supercharges circulation, improves blood flow, blood pressure and mental clarity. Nitric oxide is a natural substance produced by the body and has amazing effects on health through optimized circulation. The American Heart Association published one of many studies showing that many people over forty do not produce enough N-O. In 1998, three researchers received the Nobel Prize for its discovery. It is said there may be no disease process where N-O does not have a protective role. N-O is naturally produced by the arteries' walls. It relaxes the arteries thereby increasing blood flow to the whole body including the extremities. This increases stamina and metabolism. Our body produces less N-O as we age, so supplementation is key to staying well.

Last but not least, a comment on cosmetics. Consider this basic principle: cosmetic products should enhance one's features by working from the "inside out". For example, lipstick products that include green tea, vitamins A, C, and E, Shea butter and safflower oil will nourish your lips. Eye concealer can deliver peptides, antioxidants, proteins and age-defying ingredients such as soybean and phytosterols. Should you consider anti-aging skin care, ensure that your product of choice provides the following ingredients which make a powerful formula: resveratrol a powerful antioxidant leaves your complexion lighter; COQ10 and Vitamin E work synergistically to protect your skin from free radicals. Also, deep sea nutrients extracts promote skin elasticity and a smoother texture. It is important to know that once you take control of your health, using information of your bio-scan, there are no limits to your application of that knowledge!

In 2008, my son offered me a book entitled: *From Fatigue to Fantastic!* by Dr. Jacob Teitelbaum. That book changed my life but it took years to get there. A considerable investment of time, resources, energy went into the discovery of the root causes, professional advice on detoxification and proper supplementation to offset my fatigue. I now realize that CFS is not an "illness" in and of itself. Rather, it is a cluster of symptoms stemming from "root causes" that can vary from individual to individual. I was very fortunate to discover mine with the help of experts in the field. I will share those findings with you in my upcoming book.

Today, I wish you a super rewarding experience through this book. Follow your bio-scan, and discover why *"Wellness is Bio-Awareness"*. Visit www.biofeedbackbook.com for your initial bio-scan visit and begin your journey to health and wellness. My experience has been that if you detoxify the body from toxins and stress, the body is designed to heal itself. Unquestionably, when you are invested in your health, wellness follows very naturally!

Table 1

Cardiovascular and Cerebrovascular Data Analysis

Name: XY   Sex: Male   Age: 31
Figure: Severe partial
fat(182cm,102kg)   Testing Time: 2015-04-24 18:17

Actual Testing Results

Testing Item	Normal Range	Actual Measurement Value	Testing Result
Blood Viscosity	48.264 - 65.371	52.116	
Cholesterol Crystal	56.769 - 97.522	67.562	
Blood Fat	0.491 - 1.045	0.141	
Vascular Resistance	0.327 - 0.937	0.660	
Vascular Elasticity	1.672 - 1.978	0.662	
Myocardial Blood Demand	0.192 - 0.412	0.660	
Myocardial Blood Perfusion Volume	4.832 - 5.147	3.959	
Myocardial Oxygen Consumption	3.221 - 4.266	4.678	
Stroke Volume	1.336 - 1.672	0.926	
Left Ventricular Ejection Impedance	0.669 - 1.568	0.069	
Left Ventricular Effective Pump Power	1.556 - 1.985	0.327	
Coronary Artery Elasticity	1.552 - 2.187	1.667	
Coronary Perfusion Pressure	11.719 - 18.418	12.636	
Cerebral Blood Vessel Elasticity	0.708 - 1.942	1.316	
Brain Tissue Blood Supply Status	6.138 - 21.296	11.567	

PART TWO

CHAPTER 8
HOW STRESS DEPLETES YOUR ENERGY AND IMMUNE SYSTEM

The next three chapters allow us to move from the realm of the physical to that of the metaphysical. The first seven chapters of this book focused on the physical - the bio-awareness - aspect of health. Chapter 8 highlights stress's impact on the physical and psychological state. Chapter 9 brings to light the ramifications of destructive or toxic relationships and how to heal them. Chapter 10 threads the "connectivity" between "self-healing" and rising above the "self", in order to glimpse the "higher self's" real potential.

At this point, you[1] are likely aware of the negative impact stress has on your body and mind. Undoubtedly you have been exposed to stress and noticed, perhaps first hand, how it tenses up your muscles, accelerates your heart rate, increases blood pressure, interferes with your focus and concentration, sometimes even inducing headaches or migraines... etc. It is impossible to live stress-free. Living is stressful on your body, and science concurs. The challenge then becomes how to reduce stress in your life. We will investigate the body-mind (physiological / psychological) connection through the focus on stress-related issues, primarily those underlying "toxic" relationships. We will provide strategies to promote a "healthier you" primarily through "demystifying" common beliefs.

[1] The reader addressed in the following chapters is gender neutral. In order to facilitate the gender match between pronoun used and the subject addressed, a female personal pronoun is used. However, the "situational" context applies to either genders.

Examples of common everyday stressors abound: work; raising a family; school work; peer pressure; toxic relationships; caregiving to both your young, your elderly or to a special needs family member; financial burden; chronic illness; substance abuse or abuse of any other kind... etc. The solution is to recognize your stressors and reduce them whenever possible.

Stress and stressors are not synonymous. Stress is a stimulus, situation, behavior, condition that you face. This stimulus becomes a stressor when you "perceive" it and "categorize" it as one that is stressful to you. The situation, then, becomes a stressor for you. This is when your body responds by initializing a stress response. For example, you are driving through the rush hour period. If you perceive the drive as "stressful", then it will become a stressor causing a chain of biological and chemical reactions in your body. If, on the other hand, you categorize the tight traffic as "a normal side of living in the city", then it will not register in your brain as a stressor. By being aware that you have a choice in perceiving and categorizing a stimulus you face, you might choose to opt out of a potential stress situation. You *empower* yourself to simply switch from a stress response to, perhaps, a relaxing one, through music, relaxation technique, focusing on pleasant thoughts...etc. However, in every life span there are the inescapable stressors: losing a loved one, your home, your partner or your health...etc. This insight into your role in promoting or attenuating stressors will be determinant in your ability to reduce stress and, ultimately, cope much better with it.

How does your body respond physiologically to a stressor or stress triggers? Here is how. This is, roughly, how your brain is wired. The brain does not differentiate between "potential stress situations"[2] but merely responds to your perception and categorization of the stimulus. In the space of a 10 milliseconds, your amygdala[3] responds. The amygdala is an almond-shaped mass of nerve cell bodies, responding to danger within tens of milliseconds of detecting said danger. It is located in the center of the brain. It senses your stress perception, sends a stress response signal to the hypothalamus master gland, which relays it to the central nervous system (both sympathetic and parasympathetic). Your CNS then alerts all nerves cells centers to start producing stress hormones to prepare for an attack on the body, i.e. the stressor.

Cortisol is one example of multiple stress hormones released at the onset of stress perception. Cortisol is produced by your adrenal glands alerting your body to a "high alert" fight or flee situation. Once the stressor has dissipated, a mechanism in the body switches off the overproduction of cortisol and returns it to normal levels. However, if your stress is prolonged and becomes chronic, the mechanism is worn out and no longer is effective in controlling cortisol levels in your body. The cortisol level stays elevated constantly. This leads to adrenal fatigue due to continuous secretion of cortisol which leads you to a state of mental and physical "fatigue". This is where one appreciates clearly the mind-body connection. This is but one example of the wear and tear on your body from prolonged stress. In fact, an online search will list for you the body systems affected. They include these systems: the musculoskeletal, respiratory, cardiovascular, endocrine, gastrointestinal, nervous and both male and female reproductive system. You probably guessed by now that stress is a "toxin", a sort of "free radical" of

[2] A stressor can be potentially positive or negative and varies in its degree of intensity.

[3] The amygdala is merely one of several parts of the brain that register fear outside of our conscious awareness. For further discovery of the brain function, refer to Dr. S. S. Pillay *Life Unlocked: 7 Revolutionary Lessons to Overcome Fear*.

immeasurable consequence on your body. In fact, it is reported that 50-80% of all physical disorders have psychosomatic (psycho from the psyche; somatic through the body) stress-related origins.

Surprisingly, any emotion you feel is equally stressful for your body. For example, emotional arousal you experience occurs when any emotion, be it joy, fear, excitement, anger... etc., elicits a stress response because, at the physiological level, the brain cannot differentiate between positive and negative emotions!! For example, emotional arousal from any of the above emotions, even sexual arousal, will occur at two levels: the nervous and endocrine systems, as previously mentioned. Even a "joyful" event such as a wedding can be quite stressful. The physical, emotional and psychological demands made on the person in a short span of time (a few hours) can be overwhelming, but will largely depend on how "healthy" you are in the first place.

The *psychological* impact you feel from emotional arousal may include impaired task performance. Since stress increases your distractibility, it causes you to overthink simple tasks. The long-term impact may cause a "burnout" state. Psychological disorders such as insomnia, poor academic performance, sexual dysfunction, anxiety, depression, eating disorders... etc. are equally by-products of prolonged stress disorders.

Now that you have some understanding of the stress dynamics within your mind and body, it will be useful to you to apply strategies to enhance your coping mechanism. They are threefold: apply coping mechanisms, reduce exposure to aggravating situations, and promote a healthier you.

Coping mechanisms abound online, in self-help and stress-coping books. Exercise, meditation, neuromuscular relaxation, biofeedback and bio awareness are some of the ones most recommended. As always, apply as many coping mechanisms as possible. Buffer your odds against stress by promoting a "healthier you" (Chapter 9). Meanwhile, some more valuable strategies are available in this chapter.

The following tips may reduce your exposure to "aggravating" situations. For example, the more you surround yourself with nature (water bodies, plants, trees, beaches, mountains, fresh air…etc.), the less stressful and more energized you feel. The earth abounds with energy that you tap into when you are surrounded by its elements: water, wood, minerals, crystals, metals and stones. Feng Shui is one example of designing your home with "energy" by incorporating these energy elements into your living environment.

An essential strategy to reduce exposure to stress-related feelings such as anxiety and depression is to reduce an "emotional disconnect" between you and your loved ones. Take the initiative and "break the ice" in order to get back into "communication" mode and reconnect with the person. Communication will save any relationship even if it means the "breakup" of that relationship.

Eliminate or at least manage to cope with any form of abuse: substance abuse, physical, mental, sexual, emotional…etc. It is best to seek professional advice and guidance in doing so.

Always consider alternatives to a potentially stressful or threatening situation. For example, fear of job loss is a real stressor. You might wish to counteract that fear with information on, or the possibility of, another potential job, before you make a decision.

Working from home is now a viable alternative paradigm

for many jobs. Family can offer many blessings. An extended family member, or friends, may be a source of parental relief for you, particularly if you are a caregiver to elderly parents and children of your own. You may need to seek support from social/medical facilities, or from caregiving agencies in order to shoulder these responsibilities. Not seeking support for yourself constitutes a self-imposed unrealistic expectation which may amount to self-imposed stressors. But family can also be a source of great stressors. In today's society a "blended family", where there is integration of second marriage partners, step-children, divorce, or breakup of couples, potentially leads to stress on all members. The list of stressor possibilities in your life are specific to you and need your attention before they become chronic.

Promoting a "healthier you" is the first and last frontier. It is the one domain that should never be neglected. Looking after yourself is primarily your job. But first, let us demystify two common myths that may stand in the way of your self-wellness. The first myth is: "self-denial /self-sacrifice stands above all else". This "principle" needs to be qualified, for, as it stands, it can be very harmful to the "self". The second is: "what is familiar is normal". This notion requires equal attention to its context. It is contextual, at best, as it depends entirely on what it is you are "familiar" with.

The first myth of "self-sacrifice or denial" has been hailed as a precursor to salvation. In my view, this is an erroneous strategy. While helping others is a noble deed (see Chapter 10), it must come only after giving, or having been given, to your "self". The term "self" used here is synonymous with "being". For example, when you allow your "self" to "feel", you connect with your "being". When you neglect the self, your "self", in order to take care of others, you risk greatly damaging the one person who can effect change in yourself, in others, even in the world. That person is you.

How do you secure your "self" first? The first necessity is to love and care for yourself, and most importantly come to "like" and appreciate who you are before you can be of any service to others, even to your children. This is often misinterpreted as "selfishness". It is selfishness, only if, once you have been given, you do not give back. This is also a contextual supposition. If you grew up in a "self-sacrifice for the good of others" environment, the transition to a healthier you is more challenging since you probably learned to give others before you give yourself. This environment does not foster saying "No" to any demand or request when you really should decline to fulfill them. Nevertheless, this is a necessary step in self-awareness and it begins by discovering "who you are".

Get to know your "self", acknowledge your shortcomings and accept them for what they are, a part of you. This process can take a lifetime but you can start today. It is unquestionably worth everything. Here are some tips on how to start this process of discovering and appreciating the self in order to promote a healthier you. Be truthful with yourself and try to voice this truth to your closest allies who support you unconditionally. Sharing, in the spirit of honesty, should be mutual between you and them. Honesty is the cementing foundation of any worthwhile relationship. This honesty with yourself is the first step towards respecting your "self". Others may be inspired by your self-respect attitude towards your self and become encouraged to show you the same respect. To the best of your ability try to be truthful with others. Lies and deception lead to secrecy, feelings of guilt and fear of being discovered. These are stressful feelings. Recognize that the truth can sometimes hurt you or those you love. If so, then avoid hurting others, but at the very least, acknowledge the truth to yourself.

Psychologically, it would be very damaging for you to deny a hurtful truth from yourself. It is mentally healthy for you to live in a state of truth about your own person. Self-forgiveness, for whatever you conceive to be "wrong" or "bad", whether the act was committed by you or by others against you, is vital to self-acceptance. This is the cornerstone of self-liking. For example, imagine if someone apologized to you for a serious wrong-doing against you and you never accepted their sincere apology. Most likely, neither of you can ever go beyond the point of hurt from the wrongdoing. This applies also to you forgiving yourself. It sets you free to grow and, then perhaps, make up for the wrongdoing in some other way. The process of forgiveness allows you to heal your self. In my experience, this is the best way to love and like your self.

Allow yourself to feel. This is the strongest connection you have to your "self". Honor these feelings and never allow yourself to disconnect emotionally, or otherwise, from your "self". For example, occasionally, you may feel a certain "twinge of jealousy" towards someone, seemingly or effectively, more fortunate than you. You may simultaneously feel somewhat "guilty" for feeling this twinge of jealousy. Remember that both feelings of "jealousy" followed by "self-deprecation" are a human response, a legitimate one, so long as you do not harbor any "ill feelings or wishes" towards that person. For example, it is perfectly normal, even healthy, to wish your child would excel in a similar manner as does another classmate. There is nothing more natural than to wish the best for your child. This can be a very good motivation for you to do whatever you can to facilitate that success for your child. By focusing unto your own child, you shift your focus unto their welfare. You shift all your energy from "wishing for" into "doing for". If, alternatively, your child is not capable of such success, then as always, extend to your child a good measure of that love within you, always unconditionally, regardless of their performance. Remember that, even though feelings (negative or positive) will always raise your stress level, it is realistic to expect a relatively healthy person to cope with these feelings and dismiss them readily after they are experienced. This is why a healthy you can survive well beyond stressors in life.

"What is familiar is normal" is the second myth underlying stressful situations in life. For example, you may be drawn to an abusive relationship repeatedly. You can imagine the long-term stress incurred by your body during and after the relationship course. Usually, the person is "familiar" with the abusive behavior, it is what they "know". In fact the abuse may seem quite natural, part of life, your life. This is your "blind spot", the weak link. To cope better, you first need to know your "self". Doing so entails investigating your diverse personal traits in order to identify your "blind spot" which, necessarily at first, feels quite normal. Your only cue to investigating what seems so "normal" to you is to ask yourself two questions: "How do I feel in this relationship?" and "How is my relationship different from that of the people around me?" If, at first, you are puzzled by the "how" the relationship still survives, even if it seems abusive to you at the point of your inquiry, then, chances are, you are on your way to discovering your "blind spot". Your weak link usually feeds a pattern of behavior that puts you in a "vulnerable" position, where you may end up being hurt. This pattern becomes repetitive so long as you are unaware of its motivation. Briefly, the identifying marker of a blind spot is: a repetitive behavior which puts you at risk, by preventing you from thinking, or feeling, "any differently" about living in an unhealthy situation.

Another example of self-destructive behavior may be low self-esteem. You seek to compensate for low self-esteem by associating with people who have status, power or influence, even if they are unresponsive or worse, abusive towards you.

Again, this is where knowing your "self", your deep-seated insecurities, would be a great asset to alert you to a self-destructive behavior. For example, oftentimes, the most accomplished people have low self-esteem! As a result overachievers often "burn out" because of their overdrive to succeed. It seems almost ridiculous, until you understand the dynamics behind their undying desire to compensate for their deficit in self-esteem. This deficit may drive you to accomplish the impossible in order to gain your self-esteem. Yet, most of the "damaged" self stems from your early childhood experience. Recognition of your "accomplishments", which feeds your self-esteem as a child, should come from your parents or caregivers. It is during those tender years that your ingrained self-image becomes rooted in your psyche. If you did not experience this positive reinforcement as a child, you may spend your life trying to reverse the negative self-image by acquiring positive accolades from others, or becoming a "super achiever" at any cost.

Yet, the secret lies within "YOU". Insight into yourself has the potential to "recognize" the damage wherever it may be. Recalling how you were treated as a child helps you identify some of the issues. Ask yourself: "what were my most memorable experiences or encounters? What images or words still echo in my mind?" In my view, this investigation into your childhood is a crucial attempt to unearth the "if", the "how" and the "why" you are who you are today. It takes great courage, soul-searching, time and reflection to find your way through the past, especially if some trauma, or abuse, hinders you. Professional help may aid you to reintegrate all the parts of your "self", making you "whole" again.

CHAPTER 9
MANAGE TOXIC RELATIONSHIPS
DEPLETING YOUR MEMORY

Undoubtedly, the following is a very basic definition of what constitutes a relationship. However, this definition may help you reflect and largely determine how to qualify your relationship with the person closest to you: a life partner, a sibling, a best buddy...etc. In other words, this is someone with whom you share your day and whose input in your life matters to you. You may have more than one individual in mind; however, keep in mind that this person is the go-to person for you.

A relationship is an ongoing exchange between you and one or more individuals. The exchange can be formal, informal or intimate, as in a close relationship. The most fundamental relationships in life revolve around the need to foster support for our personal growth, thereby, hopefully, improving our quality of life. Therefore, the relationship quality is fundamental to its degree of effectiveness in supporting the person and enhancing their life.

Dr. Robert Waldinger is Director of the longest ongoing research study (1935-   ) on adult life based on the question: "What makes us happy?" His report on TedTalk (November, 2015), is a very worthwhile twelve minute video explaining why "good relationships keep us healthier and living longer". Loneliness and isolation are toxic and shorten our lives, whereas it is the "quality" of the relationship that matters to our happiness and longevity. Based on the research on 723 adults involved in the project, Dr. Waldinger affirms that good relationships protect not only our body, but our brain, where our memory stays sharper and we live longer knowing we can "count" on the other person. This is the area where you need to invest most of yourself since you stand to gain the most from good, healthy relationships.

Since relationships are the foundation of human interaction and personal fulfillment, it is imperative to foster good ones and reduce negative ones. Toxic relationships induce stress, which can affect the brain chemistry, which in turn manifests this chemical imbalance into memory loss and continuous drain on the body organs (see Chapter 8).

The effects of stress on memory have been clinically measured and medically documented; the direct relationship between stress and memory is key to this chapter. The research shows that stress interferes with a person's capacity to encode memory and the ability to retrieve information. Stress hormones, released during times of stress, can cause acute and chronic changes in certain areas of the brain causing long-term damage. At this point, suffice it to say, stress destabilizes our homeostasis or the optimum state of health that the body is capable of.

If a good relationship makes you happy, then it stands to reason that a toxic one would be a source of toxicity in your life. How do you determine whether your present relationship is toxic? The following criteria provide you with a guideline of "relationship dynamics" that support a toxic relationship. Remember that a relationship implies that more than one person is involved. Therefore, any change, positive or negative, in the existing relationship will involve you and the other person. Most importantly, there will always be at least two sides to every conflict, your side and their side.

The first part is to point out the unhealthy aspects of toxic relationships, as well as highlight tenants of strong ones. The second part reveals your role and your partner's role in "sustaining" the negative dynamics. The third part guides you in relationship-healing with strategies that can turn your relationship around, and, therefore, improve your quality of life.

The following marker can assist you in identifying toxic aspects that can be "de-toxified" if both sides work together. How does a toxic relationship feel? Common feelings in toxic relationships are feelings of rejection, rebuke, victimization and, most typically, the absence of effective communication between the parties.

Carefully note what transpires during a conflict between you and your partner. There are some very negative responses that only fuel the fire. You both should try to avoid: giving ultimatums (example "Next time I will not wait for you"). Typically, ultimatums do not leave room for discussion, negotiation, understanding, compromise, even when the person addressed is a child. Do not attempt to resolve the issue when you are in a state of anger. Emotional arousal releases stress hormones that interfere with "logical" processing of information. Keeping score of who is "right" or "wrong" only serves to distance you from one another. Blaming the other by using "blanket statements" is one sure way to sabotage your argument. For example, saying to them: "You are *always* late", as opposed to, "You are late tonight". Avoid labelling the other with what seems to be an "identification" of their "self" by using the verb "to be" (you are) in combination with a "categorical" adverb (always, never …etc.). Even the label *"lazy"* boxes the person in by most likely defeating their inclination to disprove the label, improve or change the behavior.

The most problematic underlying issue in any relationship is the absence of effective communication. Communicate frequently and effectively. For example, let your partner know in clear, calm words "how you feel when they behave in a certain way"; "what you need from them in this relationship"...etc. Never assume they already know! This sharing of your needs and goals works both ways, very effectively, when the purpose is not to rebuke a behavior or score a point, but is to bring about a change, and improve the quality of the relationship. At the very least, an acknowledgment from your partner that they now know, understand how their behavior impacts you, is a positive beginning. For example, you might have to teach them "how to love you". Usually, in a longer relationship, routine settles in and you both forget how to reach the other person who, probably, has changed over the years and, now, needs to reconfigure with you, how to go about "expressing" their love for you. To be helpful to them, ask yourself "When do I feel love(d)?", "When I am lonely or down, stressed ...etc. What do I want them to do for me to lift me up?" The answer you give may be as simple as having them: rub your feet, make your favorite drink, hold you and remain silent, clean your car inside out, ...etc. Remember women and men may differ considerably in their perception and expression of love. "Personalize" your love experience to suit you and your partner.

Another marker in a toxic relationship is that it, usually, survives under the guise of being sustained by a "noble goal". For example, one may say: "If it were not for ...the children, the family, financial burden, social or religious constraints...etc. I would not be in this relationship". There are two main motivations for staying in a failed relationship: fear or guilt. If upon examination of a troubled relationship you discover it is one or the other, or both, of these negative feelings, then at least acknowledge that fact to yourself. After the discovery of the guise you may hopefully work together towards targeting realistic, effective change. For example, should you discover that you remain in the relationship because you are afraid of living alone, then you may wish to consider rooming with a friend, a sibling...etc.

Compromise is a strong tenant, principle, of any healthy relationship. Without this vital component, any relationship is subject to failure. This is a give and take "exchange" that everyone, in a relationship, needs to practice wholeheartedly. However, there is an art to positive compromise, at the end of which you and the other person will feel "this is fair enough"! It is far less effective, if not damaging to either one, to compromise out of a sense of "obligation", "guilt" or "fear".

Understanding the mechanisms of "fair compromise" will enhance your experience of it, as well as the results you attain. Compromise requires each one of you to go beyond your comfort zone. It establishes new dimensions and guidelines for "fair exchange" between couples, or friends etc. An example might be the relationship you have with the in-law family, your partner's friends, or companions male / female, their work buddies, or even certain members of your own family ...etc. Basically, you have a "broken" relationship, or an inexistent one and you have to live with this situation.

Conflict arises when each one of you wants his way, the "whole pie" to himself. The "whole pie", as I refer to it, consists of all the elements a situation might entail, as well as your perceived "ideal way" to deal with it. Since there is always more than one person in a relationship, it stands to reason, that you may be facing a conflicting situation. Consider the following scenario. Your partner's close blood relatives may not have anything in common with you. You might find them "dull", "cheap" or "selfish"...etc. Nonetheless, your partner considers them "family", whether he agrees with you, or not, on the quality of the relationship. He strongly feels that a certain amount of "socializing" with them is necessary, even if it is not "quality socializing".

His "whole pie" could be to invite them over for dinner at your place. Your "whole pie" may be to never see them again. How do you cope? How do you make the most of a poor situation? Meaningful compromise is what it takes. Start by having a "heart-to-heart" discussion (not a fight) with your partner over your disappointment with the relationship. He may or may not agree. Regardless, he now knows how you feel. Now ask him to share how he feels. One goal is to establish together a point of interest or common concern, common ground. You establish common ground by agreeing on what each one of you can, or cannot, live with or accept. In other words, you determine together what "is" or "is not" negotiable. This is a vital departure point. For example, you both concur that "socializing" is non-negotiable, but the "how" and "where" are negotiable! That point of common ground may be the start of building together a possible compromise around how to "improvise" a new scenario for the situation at hand.

At the end of this meaningful exchange, when you have sifted through all the components of your stand and of his stand, you both should be in a position to verbalize the "negotiable" and, specifically, the "non-negotiable" components of the pending invitation. For example, his bottom line is to have a "form of socializing"; yours may be "not for dinner at our place". In order to help your partner appreciate your point of view, you may elaborate on your responsibilities as you understand them. For example, inviting people over your place is multi-tasking and burdensome for you. You work, keep house and children, look in on your elderly parent…etc. During an invite you prepare the menu, shop for items, clean house, set the table, cook the meal then get ready to "entertain". These are "components", "pieces" of the pie, which you can now propose to negotiate in order to reach a more favorable position for both of you, since you are now clear with respect to your perspective priority. A realistic compromise, or middle ground, may be to go to a restaurant, to spend a couple of hours sharing a prepared meal, while mingling without being exhausted. Remember physical exhaustion will affect your energy and focus, thus compromising your chances of being "up to" to socializing. Alternatively, you may both negotiate "shared responsibilities" for before, during and after the event. Any common agreed upon terms constitute a workable fair compromise. A compromise, if well-executed, becomes an act of sharing and healing since you should both leave with a feeling of "fairness" and even closeness in the end.

You may recall that in chapter 8 we focused briefly on examining your childhood in order to reveal what you may have "missed out on". This exercise might allow you to figure out what you have not received as a child. You may also recall that, in any relationship, reciprocity is a healthy two-way of "giving to and receiving from" the other. The above example of compromise is one application of that principle. However, you cannot give to your partner what you were not given as a child. For example, you were never encouraged to excel, to be patient, to believe in yourself, to accept your self as you are...etc. Should your partner need and / or expect these qualities from you, you would be hard-pressed to find them in you in the first place. Similarly, should your partner be unforgiving, stifling your growth, expecting you to simply acquiesce, then, chances are, he / she has learned these behaviors in their younger years and feels they are perfectly normal and good.

If you were not raised in an environment that fostered your self-acceptance, self-development and unconditional love, then you can begin to nurture yourself starting now. All you need is to decide what action you need to take to begin with. When doing so, and whenever possible, find a person(s) who support(s) your growth plan since it will necessarily mean changing. Growth comes from change. You can change and grow, providing yourself with whatever you missed out on in childhood: attention, nurturing, love, guidance, self-worth, education, a vision of who you are at your best. All you need is to draw on your inner conviction in your self as worthy of all of the above and more. This first exercise in self-growth is an excellent beginning. Now you have the strength to look into any relationship in which you feel unfulfilled.

Since life is synonymous with stress, as mentioned earlier, the issue at hand is not only to reduce your stressors (Chapter 8), but also, periodically, to monitor your stress level in order to enhance your sense of wellness. To monitor your stress level you may wish to take a four-minute questionnaire entitled *Mental Health Meter* available online (Canadian Mental Health Association). This is one amongst multiple useful tools that serves to gage your response to various stressors. Simply click on the "I agree" versus "I disagree" button. Your score is immediately given, with a guideline for its interpretation, and how to score higher. It's a relatively "engaging" exercise.

To enhance your sense of wellness, other than by healing problematic relationships, examining the self and monitoring your stress, you may wish to consider any or all of the following tips. The following self-healing tips can potentially switch your mindset, from negative to positive, allowing you to effect a change of mood. It all begins with a sense of "discovery" not only of the self, but of "visualizing" the potential of possibilities that exist beyond the self (see Chapter 10). Begin by practising *mindfulness*, a concept and a self-healing practise. It was founded by Dr. Jon Kabat-Zinn who defines the concept as a means of maintaining a "moment-by-moment awareness of your thoughts, feelings, bodily sensations, and surrounding environment". Imagine practising this technique two or three times daily to start! It can change your focus from a painful, stressful moment to one of "appreciation", for that moment, for you "being alive". You allow yourself to feel all that your body and mind can grasp from the "inside out".

Practising "daily gratitude" is a specific application of mindfulness. The gratitude concept is unique due to its multifaceted benefits. In essence, it shifts your mood, thought and focus from negative to positive since "negative" and "gratitude" are the antithesis of one another. Daily practice of "gratitude record keeping" leads to joy. A grateful you is a joyful you! You might even feel more inspired to begin this practise when you look at the *Gratitude Keeper* project inspired by Dr. Maxine Mclean. The key exercise is in reminding yourself daily to be grateful for even one event, act, word, gesture or deed, however small or insignificant it may be.

Last but not least, remember you are not alone. The universe that surrounds you responds to your attitude, your thoughts. If you are in an "attitude of gratitude", the universe will replenish your life with the same generosity of spirit, if not with much more. The film *The Secret* is an eye-opener to anyone wishing to grow beyond the self. The experts in the film advise you, the viewer, to visualize and feel intensely/vividly what you wish for. Again, they reiterate the above: daily close your eyes and feel the gratitude. Our body is the production of our thoughts. This is an extraordinary way to express the body-mind link. They reaffirm what we already discussed: disease is the result of one thing: stress, which you now may concur, is a potent toxin. Even if you should be ill, the experts in the film urge you to focus on thanking the universe (at this moment) "for your healing" (which is upcoming)! Positive thoughts or feelings continually reorganize your body.

Inspirational quotes from the experts in the film may very well resonate with you. They include: "intensely visualize whatever you wish for and it will happen gradually; man becomes what he thinks about; what you resist (negative in nature) persists; energy flows where attention goes" and, finally, "become intentional for what you want" for "inner joy allows you to attract what you want".

CHAPTER 10
SELF-ACTUALIZATION USHERS IN WELLNESS!

This chapter sheds light on the spiritual, the most mystical dimension of what I call "self-wellness", or self-actualization. In this last chapter, you shall navigate along with me the meandering paths from self-development to self-actualization. From the spiritual to the metaphysical, this chapter opens the heart and mind to free the soul.

Indeed, this final chapter is from the heart. It is greatly inspired by a lifetime of experience as daughter, sister, mother, woman, professor, writer, aunt and friend to a large family. A very enriching part of my life is due to the birth of my daughter with Down Syndrome, as well as to my struggle with Chronic Fatigue Syndrome over a period of 24 years. Counselling facilitated my struggles and energized me as I understood the nature of my struggle. My passion for research as an academic sustained me to write these life lessons which are yours to ponder today.

The title of this chapter requires two definitions: "self-actualization" and "wellness". Before we define self-actualization, you may wish to dwell, for a moment, on the composite meaning of wellness. Is it merely the cumulative effect of a healthy body and mind? Is it more than physical and mental well-being? In my view, it is infinitely more, as you shall come to find in this chapter. In fact, there are as many as eight dimensions to wellness, including occupational, social, intellectual and financial.

Ideally, self-actualization is not only the cumulative effect of a healthy body and mind, but its value exceeds the sum total of both aspects. Synergistically they combine to create the "spark", the imaginative, creative spark which motivates a person to express the self.

Consider this scenario. You may feel intangible stressors like frustration, dismay, fear, disappointment, sadness, depression, amongst many other feelings. All these feelings are a part of the majority of people's lives. You may even simultaneously experience a number of conflicting emotions that may cause you to feel overwhelmed. This would be an important moment to sift through answers as to "why" you feel this way. You possess the capability to ignite the self and allow it to cope with these stressors. You need to first allow yourself to feel them, identify them, then search within yourself for the reason(s). Remember to always be *mindful* of your state of being/feeling in the moment.

Now, reflect for a moment on this first postulate: "Life outside your self defines your existence". Ponder this second postulate for another moment: "To give of yourself to your self is personal growth", whereas, "to give of your self to others is self-actualization". It is not enough to work, earn a living or raise a family. You may need to "nourish" your self, but as in any relation (ship), you need to reciprocate, give back. If, by chance or design, you end up giving more from the plenty you feel, then you elevate yourself to a higher existence, that of a spirited, spiritual being endowed with a higher connection not only to the universe but to your soul.

Thankfully, you do not need to be perfectly healthy of body and mind to soar beyond your physical world. All you need is the "gratitude" for what you already have (specifically life itself) and the desire to be of service to your fellow man, even if it is serving, guiding others, by example only!

You question the above: "How can my service towards humanity be of any value to me?" What do "others" have to do with me?" This is a valid question in a western society where you are encouraged every day to compete and outperform others. The answer is "yes" and "no". Yes, you need to compete in order to succeed, and "no", you do not have to stop there. Once you succeed, whether partially or fully, you will wish to give back in recognition and in appreciation of those who have helped you along the way. This is your "connectivity" to humanity.

How does self-actualization unfold? In my view, self-actualization is nourished through a cause, an interest, a goal that inspires you to invest of your self into something bigger than you. All you need is simply to draw upon your strengths, your insight, your intuition and your creativity to help reach others. Your gesture of giving back allows you to feel part of the whole, of your community, of your country and of the world. This experience gives you the greatest "Dopamine hit" (the feel good hormone) that you can imagine without taking any pharmaceuticals! Without that dimension of self-actualization you could feel physically and mentally well but not passionate about anything. Day in and day out you feel no different. Perhaps, you feel vaguely disconnected from your self, or from others. Maybe the weight of the daily grind gets you down. You don't seem to have a purpose in life. You wonder what it is all about: being born, suffering, more or less, then dying. What does it all mean? You ponder the question of existentialism.

The answer, I believe, lies in being with the "higher self". Discover your higher purpose in life. In the process you will invest of yourself and your energy happily. But in doing so, you expand the horizons of the self. The process lifts you beyond the self and you feel uplifted. This process from "purpose discovery" to "self-actualization" is multi-layered.

The first stage is a *preparatory* stage. It is that of de-cluttering or resolving outstanding issues that clutter your mind, sap your energy and keep you spinning. For example, unresolved disputes, ongoing unfinished projects, outstanding debt, that need your immediate resolution; any and all are examples of what comes to mind. In resolving these you reduce the amount of "noise" in your mind, and then tune in to that inner voice, your intuitive self which nudges you softly to go beyond the self. You listen to the voice. You still don't know the "when", the "how" or the "where". But you are convinced of the "why", more so than ever before.

The second stage is the *motivational* aspect. Identify "what you love", not who you love. That which you love doing, seeing, creating, building, nourishing, growing, participating in... etc. might illuminate your vision of the next step. This stage may sound easy but it may also allude you for years. This is your bliss. Some people discover their bliss early on in life, while others find it much later. It all depends on your life journey. Regardless of the "when", it is my experience that every step you take in life is a *preparatory* one towards the realization of your call. The "how" and the "where" relate to the "nature" of the call, the time you need to grow into it. Remember, this is a lifetime journey. This is the essence of self-actualization, the meaning behind life.

The third stage is *patience*. It can go a long way here. The more you know your self, the easier you find the answer since you are now anchored in a relationship with your self. When your "juices start flowing", your energy sparkles in your eyes and the passion within you drives you to pursue what you love, chances are, you have found your call. You begin your journey towards self-actualization.

In my mind, there is a meaning to life. There is undeniably a reason for our existence. In my view, a divine plan, a higher power if you wish, is in existence. I believe that you do not necessarily discover this plan until you experience an intense, almost self-consuming desire to go beyond the self through your own "give back" need. No matter how small or insignificant a contribution you may consider, whether it is a painting for a child, a song you sing, a book you write or a kind gesture towards others...etc., all gestures/acts count as long as they are *intentional* towards connecting to others. In other words, you intend to perform the act(s) with no expected reward or recognition for yourself. This is so because helping another in any way is basically "sharing" of your self. *This is truly an act of generosity!*

The act of "giving" is multi-faceted. The act itself is communication between you and the one receiving. A strong sense of *connectedness* builds within you. The same act validates your effort to reach others in a purposeful manner. Acknowledgement for your act of giving may, or may not, be forthcoming. In fact, the less recognition you receive, the more "spiritually" elevating the act is. Nevertheless, the act has already propelled you into a greater community than your immediate one.

Examples of self-actualization are always perceived as *inspirational*. This aspect is contingent upon you, the person: "where and who you are as a person" versus "what and who you become". A vision, a feeling of that potential growth, is usually within your self. All you need is to nurture the intuitive voice within. It guides your choice of endeavour. Regardless of how ridiculous, absurd, impractical your intuitive message may seem to you, it is always worth pursuing until that endeavour of self-actualization is underway or, your intuition hints at other possibilities. This is why it is imperative to de-clutter the mind and spirit in order not to "drown" you inner voice.

The fourth stage is a *blessing*. In giving of yourself to the world, i.e. to others in the world, you sense that you are a part of the universe. How is that possible? Telecommunications, globalization and satellites have proven our physical communication. Yet, our *connectivity* has never been limited to the physical world. It is *spiritual* in essence.

The term *"spiritual"*, as referred to here, is anchored in three universal tenants: that each person is born with a body, spirit and soul; that our world encompasses physical and metaphysical dimensions; that our spiritual dimension is an expression of a higher self. Our spirit is our conduit to the beyond. This definition may, or may not, incorporate faith or religious denomination, depending on the person involved. A "spiritual" person lives in a state of consciousness of the universe and his relationship to it through his spirit and his soul.

This connectivity can also be tampered or interfered with. Much like a storm would hinder a satellite signal, your ability to connect with your soul, to the metaphysical universe, can be hindered by the "clutter". De-clutter your mind daily from the physical chores, the emotional strain, in order to hone that intuitive voice that connects you to your anchored being, and by extension, to the metaphysical realm. This is the most substantive part of your being. It has the potential to lead you to the essence of your wellness, that part of you which is eternal, your soul.

You might wonder "Is my *soul* important to my wellness? If so, why?" I have no physical measuring device to confirm or deny the presence or health-state of the soul. However, my personal journey confirms my conviction that physical and mental well-being are a reflection of the soul's state of health. More importantly, it allows you to exist beyond the self, adding a whole new dimension to life on earth.

In my view, the existence of the soul is undeniable. What is "soul"? It is that part of you that lives forever inside you and connects you to the universe. It is that part of us connected to the Supreme One, the Creator of the universe. It is that part of a human being that is holy and sacred. It is so ephemeral and yet so resilient. Its function is to nurture and sustain our humanity. It governs our deepest desires. It needs to be nurtured in order to sustain and elevate us to a higher sphere of connectivity and to all that is invisible, spiritual and metaphysical!

This book is my expression of gratitude, primarily to my Creator, and secondarily to those who sustained me along my wellness journey. It is an expression of my attempt to connect to you, my reader. To have suffered for many years for nothing is a senseless state bordering on the absurd. To have learned, through living and suffering, how to assist others in their journey effectively, is a blessing, a meaningful purpose, a gesture of "thanks and love".

www.ingramcontent.com/pod-product-compliance
Lightning Source LLC
Chambersburg PA
CBHW050539270326
41926CB00015B/3298